IOL Power Calculation Made Easy

IOL Power Calculation Made Easy

Precision at Your Fingerprints!

Editors

Jeewan S Titiyal
Chief, RP Centre & Dean (Research), AIIMS
Dr Rajendra Prasad Centre for Ophthalmic Sciences
All India Institute of Medical Sciences
New Delhi, India

Manpreet Kaur
Associate Professor
Cataract, Cornea, and Refractive Surgery Services
Dr Rajendra Prasad Centre for Ophthalmic Sciences
All India Institute of Medical Sciences
New Delhi, India

Sridevi Nair
Assistant Professor
Cataract, Cornea, and Refractive Surgery Services
Dr Rajendra Prasad Centre for Ophthalmic Sciences
All India Institute of Medical Sciences
New Delhi, India

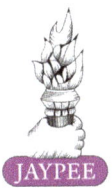

JAYPEE BROTHERS MEDICAL PUBLISHERS
The Health Sciences Publisher
New Delhi | London

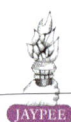 **Jaypee Brothers Medical Publishers (P) Ltd.**

Headquarters
Jaypee Brothers Medical Publishers (P) Ltd
EMCA House, 23/23-B
Ansari Road, Daryaganj
New Delhi 110 002, India
Landline: +91-11-23272143, +91-11-23272703
+91-11-23282021, +91-11-23245672
Email: jaypee@jaypeebrothers.com

Corporate Office
Jaypee Brothers Medical Publishers (P) Ltd
4838/24, Ansari Road, Daryaganj
New Delhi 110 002, India
Phone: +91-11-43574357
Fax: +91-11-43574314
Email: jaypee@jaypeebrothers.com

Overseas Office
JP Medical Ltd.
83, Victoria Street, London
SW1H 0HW (UK)
Phone: +44 20 3170 8910
Fax: +44 (0)20 3008 6180
Email: info@jpmedpub.com

Website: www.jaypeebrothers.com
Website: www.jaypeedigital.com

© 2024, Jaypee Brothers Medical Publishers

The views and opinions expressed in this book are solely those of the original contributor(s)/author(s) and do not necessarily represent those of editor(s) or publisher of the book.

All rights reserved. No part of this publication may be reproduced, stored or transmitted in any form or by any means, electronic, mechanical, photocopying, recording or otherwise, without the prior permission in writing of the publishers.

All brand names and product names used in this book are trade names, service marks, trademarks or registered trademarks of their respective owners. The publisher is not associated with any product or vendor mentioned in this book.

Medical knowledge and practice change constantly. This book is designed to provide accurate, authoritative information about the subject matter in question. However, readers are advised to check the most current information available on procedures included and check information from the manufacturer of each product to be administered, to verify the recommended dose, formula, method and duration of administration, adverse effects and contraindications. It is the responsibility of the practitioner to take all appropriate safety precautions. Neither the publisher nor the author(s)/editor(s) assume any liability for any injury and/or damage to persons or property arising from or related to use of material in this book.

This book is sold on the understanding that the publisher is not engaged in providing professional medical services. If such advice or services are required, the services of a competent medical professional should be sought.

Every effort has been made where necessary to contact holders of copyright to obtain permission to reproduce copyright material. If any have been inadvertently overlooked, the publisher will be pleased to make the necessary arrangements at the first opportunity.

Inquiries for bulk sales may be solicited at: jaypee@jaypeebrothers.com

IOL Power Calculation Made Easy: Precision at Your Fingerprints!

First Edition: **2024**

ISBN: 978-93-5696-570-6

Dedicated to

My parents, My dear wife Basanti Titiyal
My children, Dr Hemant Titiyal and Dr Renuka Titiyal
—Jeewan S Titiyal

My Alma mater and my mentors, for being the guiding light.
My family, for their unwavering support, love, and time.
—Manpreet Kaur

My teachers, for motivating me to excel.
My parents and my husband, for believing in my abilities.
—Sridevi Nair

Our patients, who constantly inspire us to perform better.
—Jeewan S Titiyal, Manpreet Kaur, Sridevi Nair

Preface

Cataract surgery is one of the most commonly performed ophthalmic surgeries worldwide and has become akin to a refractive procedure, with the patients desirous of 'perfect' outcomes after surgery.

The evolution in surgical techniques from extracapsular and intracapsular cataract extraction to microincisional sutureless phacoemulsification have been accompanied by major technological advancements in terms of sophisticated biometry devices and intraocular lens technology. A postoperative 20/20 visual acuity has become the norm, with majority of patients achieving the intended postoperative goal of near emmetropia.

Accurate biometry and IOL power calculation are the cornerstones to achieve optimal postoperative visual outcomes and patient satisfaction. The new-generation biometry devices have greatly enhanced the accuracy of measurement of various anatomical parameters. Moreover, a plethora of new generation formulae are available, which may be tailored as per the anatomical variations of the eye to further increase predictability of refractive outcomes.

This book is an endeavor to provide a comprehensive overview of different methods of estimation of ocular biometry with their pros and cons, and various IOL power calculation formulae. The salient points of each chapter are reiterated in the form of easy-to-understand flowcharts and tables, to allow the readers to grasp the significant concepts and protocols at a glance.

The book is divided into four sections sequentially covering the Evolution of IOL Power Calculation, Biometry, Present-day IOL Power Calculation Formulae and IOL Power Calculation in Challenging Situations. The highlight of this book is the section on challenging case scenarios, which will be of significant interest to all cataract surgeons, as it provides useful practical tips on how to obtain accurate biometry and which formula to use in each situation. Clinical case examples are provided at the end of each chapter with real-world case studies to further enhance understanding of the concepts.

The book is intended to serve as a comprehensive guide for all Cataract Surgeons and will be an invaluable addition to their reading list. We hope the readers enjoy perusing the book and can integrate the practical aspects to enhance their decision-making skills and clinical practice.

Jeewan S Titiyal
Manpreet Kaur
Sridevi Nair

Acknowledgments

We express our sincere gratitude to the entire staff of our Cataract Investigative Laboratories, who were of invaluable help in the meticulous maintenance of the clinical records. We gratefully acknowledge the immense efforts of the scientists, optometrists, data entry operators and research staff in ensuring comprehensive evaluation of each and every patient despite a heavy workload.

We thank all our colleagues and residents for their support. We acknowledge our patients who are an integral part of this entire venture, for placing their trust in us and providing us with an opportunity to assist them to the best of our ability.

We sincerely appreciate the entire production team of M/s Jaypee Brothers Medical Publishers (P) Ltd, New Delhi, India, for their exemplary hard-work, support, and commitment towards this project.

Contents

SECTION 1
EVOLUTION OF INTRAOCULAR LENS POWER CALCULATION

1. **Evolution of Intraocular Lens Power Calculation** 3
   - Evolution of IOL Power Calculation Formulas *3*
   - Biometry and IOL Power Calculation *5*
   - What the Future Holds *5*

SECTION 2
BIOMETRY

2. **Axial Length** 9
   - Ultrasound Biometry *9*
   - Optical Biometry *13*
   - Axial Length Measurement in Challenging Scenarios *15*

3. **Keratometry** 19
   - Methods to Calculate Corneal Power *19*
   - Instruments to Measure Corneal Power *22*
   - Corneal Power Measurement in Special Clinical Situations *29*

4. **Optical Biometry** 33
   - Types of Optical Biometers *33*
   - Optical Biometers versus Conventional Ultrasonic Methods for AL Assessment *42*
   - Comparative Evaluation of Different Optical Biometers *43*

5. **Posterior Corneal Curvature** 47
   - Defining Posterior Corneal Astigmatism *47*
   - Correlation between Anterior and Posterior Corneal Astigmatism *48*
   - Age and Posterior Corneal Astigmatism *48*
   - Measurement of Posterior Corneal Curvature *48*
   - Clinical Significance *50*

SECTION 3
INTRAOCULAR LENS POWER CALCULATION FORMULAE

6. **Regression Formulae** 57
   - Principle *57*
   - Sanders–Retzlaff–Kraff (SRK) Formula *57*

- Modifications of SRK Formula 58
- Outcomes with Regression Formulae 59
- Limitations of Regression Formulae 59
- Relevance of Regression Formulae in Current Era 59

7. Vergence Formulae 61
- Principle of Vergence Formulae 61
- Vergence Formulae 62
- Wang–Koch Adjustment in IOL Power Calculation 65
- Optimization of Intraocular Lens Constants 65
- Drawbacks of Vergence Formulae 66

8. Aberrometry-based Formulae 68
- Principle of Ray-tracing Formulae 68
- Ray-tracing Formulae 68
- Outcomes 71
- Intraoperative Aberrometry 71

9. Artificial Intelligence in Intraocular Lens Power Calculation 75
- Artificial Intelligence Methodology and Techniques 75
- Artificial Intelligence-based Intraocular Lens Power Calculation Formulae 76
- Clinical Outcomes 79
- Fallacies of Artificial Intelligence 79
- What the Future Holds 79

SECTION 4

INTRAOCULAR LENS POWER CALCULATION IN CHALLENGING SITUATIONS

10. Post-refractive Surgery Intraocular Lens Power Calculation 85
- IOL Power Calculation after Corneal Ablative Procedures 85
- IOL Power Calculation in Post-SMILE Patients 101
- IOL Power Calculation Post-Radial Keratotomy 102
- IOL Power Calculation in Phakic IOL Patients 103
- Choice of IOL 104

Clinical Case Examples 104
- Case 1 104
- Case 2 106

11. Intraocular Lens Power Calculation in Children 112
- Normal Development of the Human Eye 112
- Refractive Growth in Pseudophakic and Aphakic Pediatric Eyes 112
- Biometry 113
- Intraocular Lens Power Formula 113
- Postoperative Refractive Goal 114
- Intraocular Lens Power Calculation in Special Scenarios 116

Clinical Case Examples 117
- Case 1 117
- Case 2 117

12. Intraocular Lens Power Calculation in Corneal Pathologies 121
- Intraocular Lens Power Calculation in Corneal Ectasia *121*
- Intraocular Lens Power Calculation and Keratoplasty *127*
- Intraocular Lens Power Calculation in Corneal Scars *129*

Clinical Case Examples *129*
- Case 1 *129*
- Case 2 *130*
- Case 3 *131*

13. Intraocular Lens Power Calculation in Posterior Segment Pathology 134
- Intraocular Lens Power Calculation and Scleral Buckling *134*
- Intraocular Lens Power Calculation in Silicone-oil-filled Eyes *135*
- Intraocular Lens Power in Combined Phacovitrectomy Procedures *138*
- Intraocular Lens Power Calculation in Phacovitrectomy for Retinal Detachment *140*
- Intraocular Lens Power in Post-vitrectomized Eyes *142*

Clinical Case Examples *143*
- Case 1 *143*
- Case 2 *143*

14. Intraocular Lens Power Calculation in Extremes of Axial Length 148
- Intraocular Lens Power Calculation in Short Eyes *148*
- Intraocular Lens Power Calculation in Long Eyes (AL >26 mm) *150*

Clinical Case Examples *153*
- Case 1 *153*
- Case 2 *153*

15. Intraocular Lens Power of Piggyback IOLs and Secondary IOLs 156
- Angle-supported Anterior Chamber Intraocular Lens *156*
- Iris-fixated Intraocular Lens *157*
- Scleral-fixated Intraocular Lens *158*
- Piggyback Intraocular Lenses *158*
- Sulcus-fixated Intraocular Lens *160*

Clinical Case Examples *161*
- Case 1 *161*
- Case 2 *162*

Index 165

SECTION 1

Evolution of Intraocular Lens Power Calculation

1. Evolution of Intraocular Lens Power Calculation

CHAPTER 1

Evolution of Intraocular Lens Power Calculation

INTRODUCTION

The first intraocular lens (IOL) was implanted by Sir Harold Ridley in 1949, marking a change in the practice of ophthalmology.[1] He based his IOL power calculation on the curvature of the natural lens; however, he did not take into account the refractive index of the IOL material which resulted in refractive surprise. We have come a long way from the postoperative high residual myopia of −18 D observed with the first IOL; present-day IOL power calculation formulae help achieve a refractive accuracy within 0.5 D of the intended target in >80% of eyes, and within 1 D in >95% of eyes.[2,3]

The initial IOL power calculation formulas, or the first-generation formulas, were theoretical and regression formulas, including the original SRK I formula. Second-generation formulas included regression formulas—SRK II and modified SRK II, that modified the predicted power based on the axial length. Third-generation formulas included vergence formulas such as the Holladay 1, Hoffer Q, and SRK/T and incorporated more effective prediction of effective lens position (ELP). Newer formulas such as Barrett Universal II and Haigis incorporate multiple variables and measure anterior chamber depth (ACD) as a predictor of ELP. Ray tracing and artificial intelligence is also being used for IOL power calculation to enhance predictive accuracy and further improve refractive outcomes **(Fig. 1)**.

In this chapter, we trace the evolution of IOL power calculation formulas, from early theoretical and regression-based formulas to modern-day customized artificial intelligence (AI) based formulas.

EVOLUTION OF IOL POWER CALCULATION FORMULAS

Historical Perspective

Before the IOL power calculation formulas based on axial length and keratometry were devised, the power of the IOL to be implanted was based on the preoperative refractive status of the eye.

Early Theoretical Formulas

The initial IOL power calculation formulas were devised in 1960s to 1970s. Theoretical formulas are based on geometric optics. Fyodorov described the first theoretical formula which was based on axial length, keratometry, and calculated postoperative anterior chamber depth.[4] The formula was used for calculation of power of early anterior chamber IOLs. Other examples of first-generation theoretical formulas include the Binkhorst formula, Colenbrander formula, Thijssen's formula, Van der Heijde's formula, and Clayman's formula.

The modified Binkhorst formula is a second-generation theoretical formula that uses axial length to predict the ELP and postoperative anterior chamber depth.

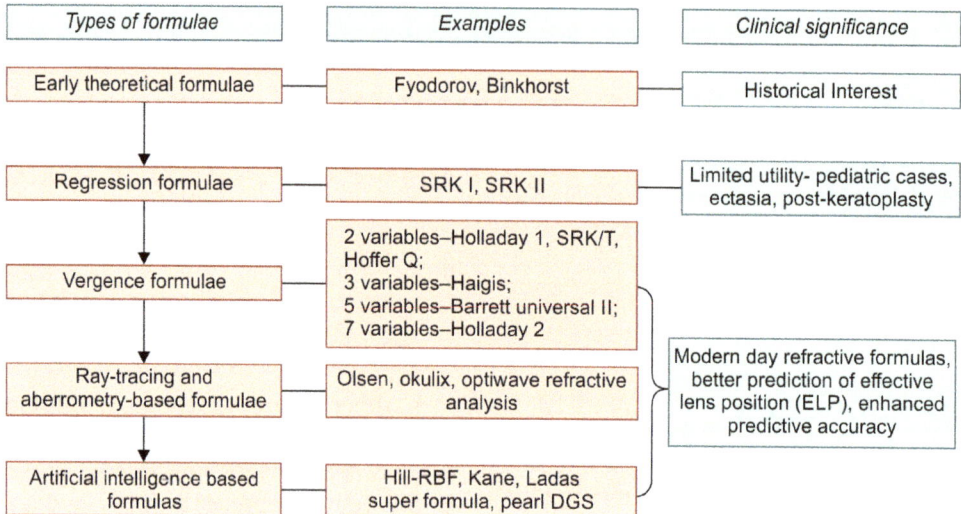

Fig. 1: Evolution of IOL power calculation formulas (IOL: intraocular lens)

These early theoretical formulas are mainly of historical interest now.

Regression Formulas

Regression formulas are based on retrospective statistical analysis of actual postoperative refractive outcomes to predict the IOL power. The original SRK formula was a regression formula devised by Donald R Sanders, John A Retzlaff, and Manus C Kraff.[5,6] The formula calculates IOL power using the equation P = A − 2.5 L − 0.9 K, where P is the IOL power, A is the IOL constant, L is the axial length, and K is the mean keratometry. The formula was fairly accurate in cases with axial length between 22 and 24.5 mm; however, there was a fall in predictability in cases with extremes of axial length.

The SRK-II formula employs correction factor for axial length and a C-value is added to the original equation of SRK I, with P = A − 2.5 L − 0.9 K + C.[7] The C-value is 3 for axial length <20 mm, 2 for axial length 20 to <21 mm, 1 for axial length 21 to <22 mm, 0 for axial length 22–24.5 mm, and −0.5 for axial length >24.5 mm. Modifications of SRK-II formula further refine the C-value to enhance refractive predictability.[8,9]

At present, SRK-I and SRK-II formulas have a limited application, usually in cases with congenital cataract that warrant on-table biometry and IOL power calculation.

Vergence Formulas

Vergence formulas are based on Gaussian optics and incorporate multiple variables to better predict the ELP. Examples of vergence formulas include the Holladay I and II formula, Hoffer Q, SRK/T, Haigis and Barrett Universal formula.[2,10] The formulas may be further classified based on the number of variables incorporated to estimate the ELP. Holladay I, SRK/T, and Hoffer Q are also known as third-generation IOL power calculation formulas and incorporate two variables to predict the ELP. Fourth-generation IOL power calculation formulas include Haigis, Barrett, and Holladay II; Haigis incorporates three variables, Barrett incorporates five, and Holladay II incorporates seven variables.

Ray-tracing and Aberrometry-based Formulas

The ray-tracing formulas take into account the corneal higher order aberrations and asphericity. Examples of ray-tracing formulas include Olsen and Okulix.[10] Optiwave refractive analysis (ORA) is an intraoperative aberrometry device that estimates IOL power based on the aphakic refraction performed by the device after phacoemulsification.

Artificial Intelligence Based Formulas

We are exploring the application of artificial intelligence (AI) in various aspects of medicine, including IOL power calculation. At present, the AI-based formulas are based on big-data and machine learning, wherein statistical algorithms are used to enhance the predictive accuracy and refine IOL power based on the analysis of large volumes of actual postoperative data. Hill-RBF is an example of pure AI-based formula; in addition, other formulas that incorporate machine learning algorithms include Ladas Super Formula 2.0, Kane and Pearl-DGS.[10-12]

BIOMETRY AND IOL POWER CALCULATION

Majority of modern day IOL power calculation formulas are based on modifications of the theoretical equation given by Fyodorov. The variables required for calculation of IOL power (P) include axial length (AL), effective lens position (ELP), desired postoperative residual refraction (R), vertex distance (V), and keratometry (K).

$$P = (1{,}336/[AL-ELP]) - (1{,}336/[1{,}336/\{1{,}000/([1{,}000/R] - V) + K\} - ELP])$$

Various devices are available to accurately measure the axial length and keratometry. ELP is predicted, taking into account various variables, and is the major limiting factor determining the predictive accuracy of various IOL power calculation formulas.

Axial Length and Keratometry Measurement

Optical biometry is the preferred method for obtaining axial length and keratometry measurements for IOL power calculation, owing to its high accuracy and predictability. Ultrasonic axial length assessment still needs to be performed in cases where optical biometry is not available or may not be captured effectively, such as pediatric patients, uncooperative patients with poor fixation, dense cataract, etc.

Posterior corneal curvature is measured by majority of newer keratometry devices and should be accounted for to obtain total keratometry values.

Effective Lens Position

Accurately predicting the ELP is increasingly recognized as the key to achieving precise refractive outcomes after cataract surgery. Modern-day biometry devices enable precise axial length and keratometry measurements; however, reliably predicting the ELP in every case still remains a challenge.

The first-generation theoretical formulas used a fixed value of anterior chamber depth to calculate IOL power. Further generations of IOL power calculation formulas scaled the ELP based on axial length (second-generation formulas), axial length and keratometry (third-generation formulas), or multiple variables including lens thickness, white to white, preoperative anterior chamber depth, etc. (fourth-generation formulas) **(Table 1)**.

Ray tracing and artificial intelligence algorithms are now being used to enhance the predictive accuracy of ELP and IOL power formulas.[13]

WHAT THE FUTURE HOLDS

The early theoretical and regression-based formulas are mainly of historical interest. Present-day IOL power calculation formulas include the multiple-variable vergence formulas, ray tracing formulas, and AI-based formulas. The advancement in IOL power calculation formulas relies on sophisticated

TABLE 1: Estimation of effective lens position with different generations of IOL power formulae

IOL power formula	Estimation of effective lens position
First-generation formulas	Fixed value—4.5 mm
Second-generation formulas	*Scaling of ELP based on axial length:* • Axial length 10% longer than average—use value 10% greater than 4.5 mm to calculate ELP • Axial length 10% smaller than average—use value 10% shorter than 4.5 mm to calculate ELP
Third-generation formulas	Scaling of ELP based on two variables—axial length and keratometry
Fourth-generation formulas	Multiple variables used to predict ELP, including axial length, keratometry, preoperative ACD, LT, WTW, etc.
Modern-day formulas	Ray tracing and AI algorithms incorporated in prediction of ELP

(ACD: anterior chamber depth; AI: artificial intelligence; ELP: effective lens position; IOL: intraocular lens; LT: lens thickness; WTW: white to white)

biometry acquisition devices. We have moved forward from ultrasonic axial length estimation and placido disk-based keratometers to modern-day biometers, which have become the current benchmark for obtaining the axial length and keratometry measurements. In addition, the biometers account for posterior corneal curvature to further enhance the predictive accuracy. With continuous fine-tuning of various formulas and incorporation of machine-learning algorithms, it may be feasible to achieve a refractive outcome within 0.5 D of intended target in >95% of cases.

REFERENCES

1. Apple DJ, Sims J. Harold Ridley and the invention of the intraocular lens. Surv Ophthalmol. 1996;40:279-92.
2. Melles RB, Kane JX, Olsen T, Chang WJ. Update on Intraocular Lens Calculation Formulas. Ophthalmology. 2019;126:1334-5
3. Melles RB, Holladay JT, Chang WJ. Accuracy of Intraocular Lens Calculation Formulas. Ophthalmology. 2018;125:169-78.
4. Fyodorov SN, Galin MA, Linksz A. Calculation of the optical power of intraocular lenses. Invest Ophthalmol. 1975;14:625-8.
5. Sanders DR, Kraff MC. Improvement of intraocular lens power calculation using empirical data. J Am Intra Ocul Implant Soc. 1980;6:263-7.
6. Retzlaff J. A new intraocular lens calculation formula. J Am Intra Ocul Implant Soc. 1980;6:148-52.
7. Sanders DR, Retzlaff J, Kraff MC. Comparison of the SRK II formula and other second generation formulas. J Cataract Refract Surg. 1988;14:136-41.
8. Dang MS, Raj PP. SRK II formula in the calculation of intraocular lens power. Br J Ophthalmol. 1989;73:823-6.
9. Kora Y, Suzuki Y, Inatomi M, Ozawa T, Fukado Y. A simple modified SRK formula for severely myopic eyes. Ophthalmic Surg. 1990;21:266-71.
10. Xia T, Martinez CE, Tsai LM. Update on Intraocular Lens Formulas and Calculations. Asia Pac J Ophthalmol. 2020;9:186.
11. Kane JX, Van Heerden A, Atik A, Petsoglou C. Accuracy of 3 new methods for intraocular lens power selection. J Cataract Refract Surg. 2017;43:333-9.
12. IOL Power Calculator for Cataract Surgery. Hill-RBF Calculator. [online] Available from https://rbfcalculator.com/. [Last accessed January, 2024].
13. Li T, Stein J, Nallasamy N. AI-powered effective lens position prediction improves the accuracy of existing lens formulas. Br J Ophthalmol. 2022;106:1222-6.

SECTION 2

Biometry

2. Axial Length
3. Keratometry
4. Optical Biometry
5. Posterior Corneal Curvature

CHAPTER 2

Axial Length

■ INTRODUCTION

Accurate biometry is a prerequisite for precise intraocular lens (IOL) power calculation. Axial length (AL) assessment is the most significant aspect of preoperative biometry, with an error of 0.1 mm in AL measurement associated with nearly 0.28 diopters (D) of postoperative residual refractive error.[1] Inaccuracies in AL assessment contribute to 17–54% of the post-cataract surgery residual refractive errors.[2,3] Conventionally, ultrasonic biometry was used for assessment of AL using either contact or immersion methods, with an accuracy ranging from ±0.05 to ±0.1 mm. Optical biometry methods have enhanced the precision of AL measurement to ±0.02 mm and are the preferred modality at present; however, ultrasonic methods still retain their significance in cases wherein optical biometry methods are not feasible. In this chapter, we discuss various methods of AL measurement and their specific application in various challenging case scenarios.

■ ULTRASOUND BIOMETRY

Ultrasonic biometry or A-scan biometry measures the anatomical AL from the corneal vertex up to the internal limiting membrane. An "amplitude" or "A" scan is typically used to measure the AL, wherein high-frequency sound waves penetrating the eye get reflected towards the probe on encountering a media interface.

Principle

Measurements using ultrasound biometry are based on the time taken for the sound waves to travel from one point to another. The formula "Distance = Velocity × Time" is used, and the time taken for the echoes to return to the probe is used to determine the distance between the probe and the various ocular structures, with the amplitude of reflected sound represented by the height of spikes on a visual monitor.[4] Typically, a 10-MHz ultrasound transducer or probe is used which has a longitudinal resolution of about 200 microns.[5]

Techniques of Ultrasound Biometry

Axial length may be determined by either the contact method or immersion method. The contact or applanation technique involves a direct contact between the ultrasonic probe and the cornea. Immersion technique involves the use of a fluid coupling media while avoiding direct corneal contact, has a higher accuracy, and is the conventional gold standard for AL estimation.[6]

Pre-measurement Considerations

Axial length measurements are obtained after instilling topical anesthesia in the patient's eyes. Keratometry readings should be obtained prior to AL acquisition. Before performing the procedure, the A-scan probe is cleaned with a damp gauze pad. In cases undergoing immersion scan, the scleral shell is disinfected using alcohol or hydrogen peroxide. The appropriate acquisition mode (manual or automatic), the technique (contact or immersion), and status of the eye (phakic, aphakic, or pseudophakic) should be selected.

Contact Technique

Applanation biometry, or contact biometry, may be performed with the patient seated or in supine position, using a hand-held or a slit-lamp mounted probe. The patient is instructed to look into the probe tip fixation light which is then gently touched upon the cornea. Care should be taken to hold the probe perpendicular to the cornea while avoiding any indentation **(Fig. 1)**.[7]

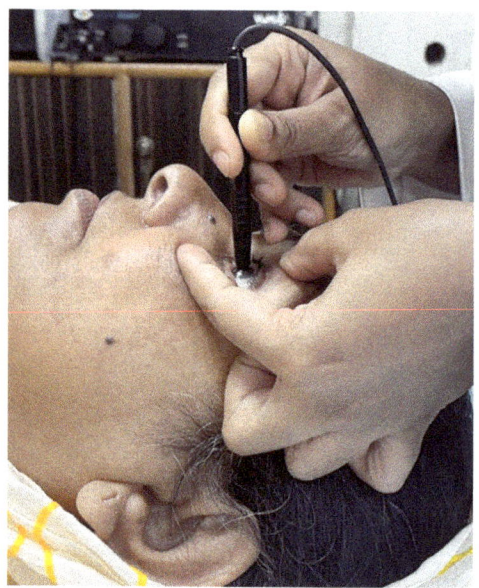

Fig. 1: Contact A-scan being performed while the patient looks up into the probe tip fixation light, with the probe gently touching the cornea

Immersion Technique

The patient is placed supine with eyes in the primary gaze. An open scleral shell (Ossoinig or Hansen scleral shells) with a routine A-Scan probe is commonly employed; alternatively, a fixed immersion shell (Prager shell) with attached tubing for fluid infusion and a mounted probe may be used **(Fig. 2)**. The scleral shell is placed beneath the lids and filled with a coupling media such as normal saline or hydroxypropyl methylcellulose. The ultrasound probe is held within the fluid, without touching the cornea. The tubing of the Prager shell should be discarded after each use.[8]

Contact versus Immersion Technique

Comparative evaluation of methods, accuracy, advantages, and limitations of contact and immersion methods of ultrasound biometry is summarized in **Table 1**.

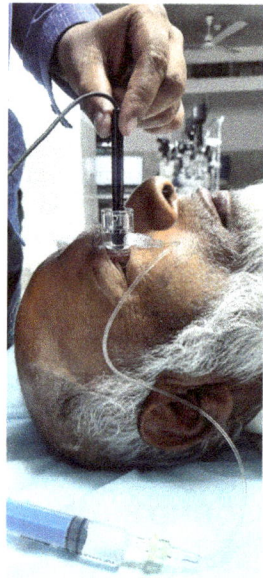

Fig. 2: An immersion A-scan being performed using a Prager shell

The contact A-scan has a precision of ±0.1 mm.[9] It is more widely performed as it is convenient and less time-consuming.

TABLE 1: Techniques of ultrasonic biometry for axial length estimation

	Contact technique	Immersion technique
Technique	• Contact method • Ultrasound probe directly touched to corneal surface	• Noncontact method • Probe suspended in fluid-filled scleral shell
Precision	±0.1 mm	±0.05 mm
Advantage	Easy, convenient, fast	• More precise • No corneal indentation
Limitation	Corneal indentation by probe—false low axial length reading (0.14–0.47 mm shorter)	• Cumbersome, time consuming • Risk of infection by contaminated scleral shell or tubings

BOX 1: Characteristics of a good A-scan

- Five steeply rising spikes of equal height corresponding to the probe tip or cornea, anterior and posterior lens capsule, retina, and sclera
- Orbital fat echo pattern, denoted by a series of highly reflective spikes, seen posterior to the retinal and scleral spike
- Deepest anterior chamber measurement—associated with the least corneal compression
- Thickest lens measurement—ensures ultrasound beam directed nearest to center of the lens
- Gain of 70–75%
- *Correct mode and velocity:* Phakic/pseudophakic/aphakic/oil-filled

The direct contact of the probe with the cornea may result in inadvertent corneal indentation with underestimation of the true AL. Moreover, the varying degrees of compression result in wider variability of measurements.

The immersion technique does not cause corneal indentation, is more reproducible, and has a greater precision of ±0.05 mm. AL obtained with immersion technique is approximately 0.14–0.47 mm longer as compared with that obtained using a contact A-scan.[6] Immersion biometry can measure the AL through any axial opacity, including dence cataracts. On the flip side, the shell and tubing used in immersion biometry may be a source of microbial contamination of the ocular surface.

Interpreting the A-scan

A good quality A-scan is characterized by five steeply rising spikes of equal height corresponding to the probe tip or cornea, anterior and posterior lens capsule, retina, and sclera **(Box 1 and Fig. 3)**. The orbital fat echo pattern, denoted by a series of highly reflective spikes, should be identified posterior to the retinal and scleral spike. This confirms that the scan is through the macula and not the optic nerve head. Multiple scans are acquired and the average value of 3–5 good quality scans is commonly used. A good scan preferably includes the deepest anterior chamber measurement as it is associated with the least corneal compression. Selecting a scan with the thickest lens measurement helps to ensure that the ultrasound beam was directed nearest to the center of the lens. Stair-stepped poorly formed spikes or low amplitude spikes are indicative of poor alignment with the visual axis and the scan should preferably be repeated. The distance between the two spikes may be measured using electronic calipers known as 'gates'. Ideally, gates are placed on the ascending edge of the spikes for accurate measurement. Conventionally, four gates are placed corresponding to the cornea, anterior lens surface, posterior lens surface and retina. The velocity of the ultrasonic beam varies based on the structure between the two gates;

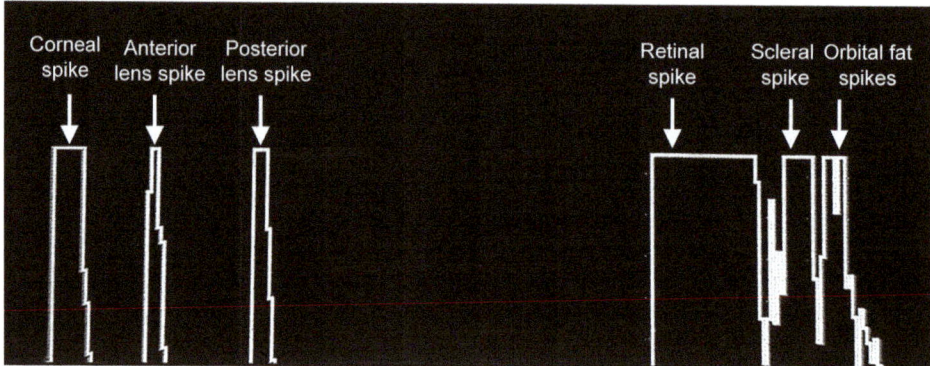

Fig. 3: A good quality A-scan depicting five steeply rising spikes of equal height

for example, 1,532 m/s between first and second gate (anterior chamber), 1,641 m/s between second and third gate (lens), and 1,532 m/s between third and fourth gate (vitreous cavity) in a phakic eye. The gates are placed automatically in most ultrasonic biometers and the accuracy of their alignment should be checked; some devices may allow manual adjustment of the position of the gates.

The electronic amplification factor or "gain" is normally set at about 70–75%. It may, however, be increased in cases with dense cataract, corneal opacities, or high myopia. Keeping the gain too high may lead to merging of retinal and scleral spikes. Flattening of the top of spikes may be observed if the amplitude gain is too high, which results in inaccurate measurements.

Correct velocity must be selected while performing an ultrasonic A-scan. The average velocity is 1,550 m/s for the phakic eye and 1,532 m/s for the aphakic eye. In pseudophakia, the velocity depends on the IOL material and a correction factor may be added to the axial length obtained using aphakic mode based on the type of IOL (+0.4 mm for PMMA IOL, +0.2 mm for acrylic IOL, –0.4 to –0.8 mm for silicone IOL).

The use of supplemental 2-dimensional B-scan may be helpful in scenarios such as posterior staphyloma and retinal detachment, as it allows the operator to direct the AL measurement to the region of the fovea. B-scan may also be performed if an unusual spike is observed during A-scan to rule out an abnormal lesion in the eye.

Sources of Error in Ultrasound Biometry

Accurate AL measurement is essential for precise IOL power calculation and optimal visual outcomes. Ensuring the correct measurement technique is the key to achieve good results with ultrasound biometry. Several sources of errors may result in fallacies of AL measurement and postoperative refractive surprise **(Table 2)**.

- *Corneal indentation:* Corneal compression during a contact A-scan can lead to false low estimate of AL. A 0.4-mm compression will result in nearly 1D error in the calculated IOL power. The refractive consequence of AL underestimation is more pronounced in shorter eyes.[10]
- *Misalignment of ultrasound beam:* Parallax difficulties in centering the probe may be observed, especially while performing a contact A-scan. If the probe is not perpendicular to the lens or macula, a poor lens or retinal spike may be observed.

TABLE 2: Limitations and sources of error in A-scan ultrasound biometry

Source of error	Impact on measurement
Gain too high	• Flattening of spikes • Merging of retinal and scleral spikes
Misaligned beam	• Low amplitude spikes—decrease in amplitude with increase in angulation of probe • Absence of orbital fat echoes indicates scan through optic nerve head
Incorrect velocity	• Too short or long measurements obtained if correct mode not selected • Axial length in pseudophakia = Axial length in aphakic mode (1,532 m/s) + correction factor for IOL material (+0.4 mm for PMMA, +0.2 mm for acrylic, −0.4 to −0.8 mm for silicone, depending on silicone velocity)
Corneal indentation	0.4 mm compression leads to 1 D error in IOL power

(IOL: intraocular lens)

Absence of scleral spike or orbital fat echoes is suggestive of misalignment with the scan obtained along the optic nerve. False high reading may be observed in cases of posterior staphyloma or by measuring the scleral spike instead of retinal spike.[11]

- *Incorrect velocity:* Incorrect sound velocity can result in false low or high readings. If the eye is not phakic, it is important to change the setting, so the machine uses the correct velocity for either an aphakic, pseudophakic, or silicone oil filled eye. An assumption of constant ultrasound speed is made for each structure within the eye; however, the acoustic properties of the eye structures may considerably differ. For example, the acoustic properties inside the lens may vary significantly for diverse cataract types and severities.[12]
- *Limited axial resolution attained at 10 MHz:* This limitation can affect the correct identification of the retinal-choroid interface because of the small thickness of these structures.

OPTICAL BIOMETRY

Optical biometry is a noncontact modality which uses an infrared laser source to measure AL. It is the current gold standard in AL measurement.

The two major limitations with ultrasound biometry are that it measures the anatomical AL from corneal vertex to the posterior pole of the eye, which is longer than the optical AL measured along the visual axis of the eye passing through fovea. This error is magnified in eyes with AL longer than 26 mm. Secondly, ultrasound biometry measures the AL from corneal surface to internal limiting membrane, and not till the photoreceptor layer located near the back of the retina. An average retinal thickness of 200 microns was incorporated in older IOL power calculation formulas to obtain corrected AL; however, retinal thickness varies from 160 to 400 microns which may lead to fallacies in IOL power calculation. Optical biometers measure the true optical AL and address the limitations observed with ultrasound biometry.

Principle

Initial optical biometers were based on the principle of partial coherence interferometry (PCI) or optical low coherence reflectometry (OLCR). Now, swept source optical coherence tomography (SS-OCT) based optical biometers are increasingly being used in clinical practice due to their enhanced precision and accuracy. The newer SS-OCT-based optical biometers have several advantages over the conventional PCI devices including short scan-acquisition time, less motion artifacts, deeper tissue penetration, and high axial resolution. These devices also allow the accurate assessment of fixation status by visualization of fovea on the macular OCT image. Types of optical biometers, their principles, and clinical applications are discussed in detail in Chapter 4.

Technique

The patient fixates on a target light, and optical biometers measure the AL from the tear film to the retinal pigment epithelium along the visual axis.[13] On average, the AL measurements obtained by contact ultrasound are 20–390 microns shorter, and those obtained by immersion ultrasound are 40–87 microns shorter as compared with optical biometry.[14-16] The variability may be attributed to the corneal indentation in contact ultrasound method, as well as the difference in the measuring points of the techniques. The optical biometers incorporate a software that calibrates the optically measured AL against the value measurable by the immersion ultrasound technique.[17] **Table 3** compares the characteristics of ultrasound biometry and optical biometry.

Advantages

Optical biometers have a higher accuracy of ±0.02 mm and less variability as compared with ultrasound biometry and are the preferred modality in present-day practice for AL estimation.[18] They measure the true optical AL from the corneal vertex to the fovea.

Limitations

A major limitation of the laser interferometry based optical biometers is their inability to successfully measure the AL in dense nuclear and posterior subcapsular cataracts, with a reported failure rate ranging from 4.7 to 37.8%.[5,19] The incorporation of SS-OCT technology for AL measurement has largely mitigated this problem. The higher wavelength (1,055 nm) used in SS-OCT technology results in less scattering with better penetration, with only 1% scans unable to successfully capture the AL.[20]

TABLE 3: Comparative evaluation of ultrasound and optical biometry for axial length estimation

Ultrasound biometry	Optical biometry
Uses sound waves to measure axial length	Uses infrared laser beam to measure axial length
• Contact A-scan requires corneal contact with probe • Risk of infection and corneal abrasion	Noncontact method
Measures AL along anatomic axis—from cornea to internal limiting membrane	Measures AL along visual axis—from tear film to retinal pigment epithelium
Uses segmental measurements with individual sound velocities for different components of the eye	Most devices use a mean group optical refractive index
Lower accuracy (±0.1–0.05 mm), higher variability	Higher accuracy (±0.02 mm), lower variability
Can be performed under general anesthesia	• Requires patient to fix on the light source • Not suitable for uncooperative patients, patients with nystagmus or under general anesthesia
Requires a trained, experienced observer	Less operator dependent

(AL: axial length)

Optical biometers require the patient to fixate on the fixation light during scan acquisition. Therefore, it is not suitable for pediatric patients where biometry is acquired during examination under anesthesia. In addition, reliable scan acquisition may not be feasible in uncooperative patients, patients with nystagmus, or inability to fixate.

AXIAL LENGTH MEASUREMENT IN CHALLENGING SCENARIOS

Accurate measurement of AL in certain clinical scenarios can be challenging. These include cases of retinal detachment, vitreoretinal pathologies, posterior staphyloma, and silicone oil filled eyes. **Table 4** highlights the difficulties faced during AL estimation in challenging scenarios along with the preferred technique.

Retinal Detachment

Combined phacoemulsification and pars plana vitrectomy may be required in cases of retinal detachment with a significant cataract. Erroneous results in macula-off retinal detachment are attributed to poor fixation by the patient and a false low AL reading due to anterior displacement of the vitreoretinal interface, which may interfere with the sound waves or light signals. In eyes with large detachments where AL cannot be acquired with optical biometers, an immersion A-scan may provide a less erroneous result as the height of RD reduces in the supine position. A combined vector-A/B-scan which helps in direct visualization of foveal location may also be a useful method in these cases.[21] In optical biometry, if the posterior peak corresponds to the detached retina, a manual adjustment to shift the signal peak selection

TABLE 4: Axial length estimation in challenging case scenarios

Special scenario	Challenge	Preferred method
Dense cataract	Infrared beam may not penetrate dense cataract	Immersion ultrasound. SS-OCT may be useful in some cases
Retinal detachment	Anteriorly located detached retina interferes with sound and light signals producing false low AL readings	• Optical biometry, especially the SS-OCT-based devices • Immersion A-scan or combined vector-A/B-scan if AL cannot be measured using optical methods
Silicone oil (SiO) filled eyes	• Speed and refractive index of SiO differs from that of vitreous • SiO has sound and light attenuating properties • Incomplete fill, oil droplet artefacts	• Optical biometry preferred • In cases of dense cataract where optical biometry is not feasible, immersion A-scan should be performed
Posterior staphyloma	Depth of staphyloma measured with ultrasound rather than fovea due to misalignment from the visual axis	Optical biometry which measures AL along visual axis. SS-OCT-based devices more accurate as they allow direct visualization of fixation status
Vitreoretinal interface abnormalities	Anterior displacement of vitreoretinal interface—AL significantly smaller when measured with ultrasound A-scan	Optical biometry preferable—less affected by retinal thickening. In case of double peak, posterior peak should be used

(AL: axial length; SS-OCT: swept source optical coherence tomography)

to a more posterior peak with an SNR of 2 dB or more can be performed.[22] If reliable values cannot be obtained with any method, fellow eye AL may be used as a last resort, provided the refractive error between the two eyes is comparable.

Vitreoretinal Interface Abnormalities

Axial length measurement in cases of vitreoretinal interface pathologies such as macular edema, epiretinal membrane (ERM), and vitreomacular traction (VMT) is prone to errors owing to increased thickness of the retina or highly reflective membranes at vitreoretinal interface. Optical biometry is more accurate in these cases as compared to ultrasound biometry. While measuring the AL using optical biometers, a double peak may be observed in cases of macular edema or ERM and the use of posterior peak which denotes the RPE is recommended for AL estimation.[23,24] SS-OCT-based biometers give more accurate results in cases of vitreoretinal interface abnormalities as compared to partial coherence interferometry (PCI) based devices.[24]

Posterior Staphyloma

In posterior staphyloma, the AL can be erroneously longer if the depth of the staphyloma is measured rather than the fovea, often due to inaccurate fixation or misalignment during measurement. Optical biometry is preferred for these cases. SS-OCT-based devices provide a more accurate AL measurement in these eyes as it allows the evaluation of fixation status based on the macular OCT image which should ideally include the foveal pit **(Fig. 4)**.[25]

Silicone Oil-filled Eyes

Obtaining accurate AL measurement in silicone oil-filled eyes can be challenging. Silicone oil has a different refractive index than vitreous which alters the speed of both sound and light waves within the medium resulting in an erroneously longer AL.

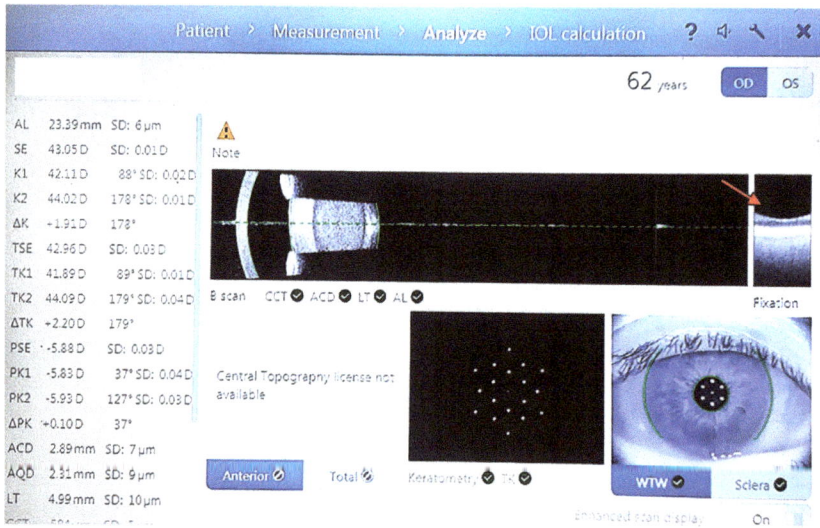

Fig. 4: AL-scan acquired using SS-OCT optical biometer (IOLMaster 700). Fixation status can be confirmed by identifying the foveal pit on the macular OCT image (red arrow) (AL: axial length; SS-OCT: swept source optical coherence tomography)

It also has optical and sound attenuation properties which adversely impacts the AL measurement. Optical biometry is more accurate for AL estimation in oil-filled eyes. These devices are calibrated to automatically adjust for the difference in refractive index. However, errors in optical biometry can occur if the vitreous cavity is underfilled, or due to oil droplet artifacts. Moreover, cataracts in oil-filled eyes are often dense and a significant rate of measurement failure of up to 26% has been observed with PCI-based devices.[26]

Ultrasound biometry is an alternative in these cases with immersion technique being preferred over contact method. While performing an A-scan in an oil-filled eye, the speed of sound through vitreous cavity needs to be adjusted (987 m/s in 1,000 cS viscosity silicone oil). If the device does not permit speed adjustment, a conversion factor (0.71 for 1,300 cS and 0.64 for 1,000 cS silicone oil) can be multiplied to the measured vitreous cavity length which is then added to the length of remaining segments, namely lens thickness and anterior chamber depth to estimate the corrected AL. An incomplete oil fill is an important source of error in AL estimation as it results in a retro-silicone oil space when patient is lying in the supine position. This fluid-filled space has the same velocity as that of vitreous which should be ideally factored in while computing the AL. An immersion B-scan guided biometry can aid in identification of ocular interfaces including a retro-silicone space.[27]

■ CONCLUSION

Accurate AL measurement is one of the prerequisites for achieving optimal refractive outcomes after cataract surgery. Ultrasound biometry remains a widely used technique for AL estimation, with immersion technique having greater accuracy and reproducibility as compared with contact technique. Optical biometry is noninvasive, easier to perform and more accurate and has arguably become the current gold standard for AL estimation. However, ultrasound biometry may still be required in cases with dense cataracts precluding scan acquisition using optical biometry. Pediatric patients, uncooperative patients with poor fixation or nystagmus also require ultrasound biometry for AL measurement. Axial length assessment in challenging scenarios should be performed carefully and the use of more than one modality may be required for accurate AL estimation.

■ REFERENCES

1. Olsen T. Theoretical approach to intraocular lens calculation using Gaussian optics. J Cataract Refract Surg. 1987;13(2):141-5.
2. Olsen T. Sources of error in intraocular lens power calculation. J Cataract Refract Surg. 1992;18(2):125-9.
3. Norrby S. Sources of error in intraocular lens power calculation. J Cataract Refract Surg. 2008;34(3):368-76.
4. Shammas HJ. Axial length measurement and its relation to intraocular lens power calculations. J Am Intraocul Implant Soc. 1982;8(4):346-9.
5. Rajan MS, Keilhorn I, Bell JA. Partial coherence laser interferometry vs conventional ultrasound biometry in intraocular lens power calculations. Eye (Lond). 2002;16(5):552-6.
6. Hennessy MP, Franzco, Chan DG. Contact versus immersion biometry of axial length before cataract surgery. J Cataract Refract Surg. 2003;29(11):2195-8.
7. Shammas HJ. A comparison of immersion and contact techniques for axial length measurement. J Am Intraocul Implant Soc. 1984;10(4):444-7.
8. Watson A, Armstrong R. Contact or immersion technique for axial length measurement? Aust N Z J Ophthalmol. 1999;27(1):49-51.

9. Freudiger H, Artaria L, Niesel P. Influence of intraocular lenses on ultrasound axial length measurement: in vitro and in vivo studies. J Am Intraocul Implant Soc. 1984;10(1):29-34.
10. Shroff NM, Ray S, Dutta, Kumar K. A practical device to aid in immersion a-scan biometry. J Cataract Refract Surg. 2004;30(6):1386-7.
11. Astbury N, Ramamurthy B. How to avoid mistakes in biometry. Community Eye Health. 2006;19(60):70-1.
12. Petrella L, Perdigão F, Caixinha M, Santos M, Lopes M, Gomes M, et al. A-scan ultrasound in ophthalmology: A simulation tool. Med Eng Phys. 2021;97:18-24.
13. Németh J, Fekete O, Pesztenlehrer N. Optical and ultrasound measurement of axial length and anterior chamber depth for intraocular lens power calculation. J Cataract Refract Surg. 2003;29(1):85-8.
14. Attas-Fox L, Zadok D, Gerber Y, Morad Y, Eting E, Benamou N, et al. Axial length measurement in eyes with diabetic macular edema: a-scan ultrasound versus IOLMaster. Ophthalmology. 2007;114(8):1499-504.
15. Cooke DL, Waldron R, Savini G, Riaz KM, Taroni L, Murphy DA, et al. Immersion ultrasound biometry vs optical biometry. J Cataract Refract Surg. 2022;48(7):819-25.
16. Goyal R, North RV, Morgan JE. Comparison of laser interferometry and ultrasound A-scan in the measurement of axial length. Acta Ophthalmol Scand. 2003;81(4):331-5.
17. Haigis W, Lege B, Miller N, Schneider B. Comparison of immersion ultrasound biometry and partial coherence interferometry for intraocular lens calculation according to Haigis. Graefes Arch Clin Exp Ophthalmol. 2000;238(9):765-73.
18. Lee AC, Qazi MA, Pepose JS. Biometry and intraocular lens power calculation. Curr Opin Ophthalmol. 2008;19(1):13-7.
19. McAlinden C, Wang Q, Pesudovs K, Yang X, Bao F, Yu A, et al. Axial Length Measurement Failure Rates with the IOLMaster and Lenstar LS 900 in Eyes with Cataract. PLoS ONE. 2015;10(6):e0128929.
20. Hirnschall N, Varsits R, Doeller B, Findl O. Enhanced Penetration for Axial Length Measurement of Eyes with Dense Cataracts Using Swept Source Optical Coherence Tomography: A Consecutive Observational Study. Ophthalmol Ther. 2018;7(1):119-24.
21. Abou-Shousha M, Helaly HA, Osman IM. The accuracy of axial length measurements in cases of macula-off retinal detachment. Can J Ophthalmol. 2016;51(2):108-12.
22. Rahman R, Kolb S, Bong CX, Stephenson J. Accuracy of user-adjusted axial length measurements with optical biometry in eyes having combined phacovitrectomy for macular-off rhegmatogenous retinal detachment. J Cataract Refract Surg. 2016;42(7):1009-14.
23. Kojima T, Tamaoki A, Yoshida N, Kaga T, Suto C, Ichikawa K. Evaluation of axial length measurement of the eye using partial coherence interferometry and ultrasound in cases of macular disease. Ophthalmology. 2010;117(9):1750-4.
24. Faraldi F, Lavia CA, Nassisi M, Kilian RA, Bacherini D, Rizzo S. Swept-source OCT reduces the risk of axial length measurement errors in eyes with cataract and epiretinal membranes. PLoS One. 2021;16(9):e0257654.
25. Yang JY, Kim HK, Kim SS. Axial length measurements: Comparison of a new swept-source optical coherence tomography-based biometer and partial coherence interferometry in myopia. J Cataract Refract Surg. 2017;43(3):328-32.
26. Nepp J, Krepler K, Jandrasits K, Hauff W, Hanselmayer G, Velikay-Parel M, et al. Biometry and refractive outcome of eyes filled with silicone oil by standardized echography and partial coherence interferometry. Graefes Arch Clin Exp Ophthalmol. 2005;243(10):967-72.
27. Abu El Einen KG, Shalaby MH, El Shiwy HT. Immersion B-guided versus contact A-mode biometry for accurate measurement of axial length and intraocular lens power calculation in siliconized eyes. Retina (Philadelphia, PA). 2011;31(2):262-5.

CHAPTER 3

Keratometry

■ INTRODUCTION

Keratometry refers to the measurement of corneal curvature and power, and is one of the essential parameters required for intraocular lens (IOL) power calculation. A 1 diopter (D) error in keratometry is associated with a nearly 1D error in IOL power calculation.[1]

Hermann von Helmholtz is credited with devising the first keratometer for clinical use in 1851.[2] Conventional keratometry devices measure the anterior corneal curvature alone and assume a fixed relationship between anterior and posterior corneal curvature to determine corneal power. Optical biometry and corneal tomography devices have enhanced the precision of corneal power measurements; most new-generation devices directly measure both anterior and posterior corneal curvature, are more accurate, and have increased applicability in conditions where the normal cornea is altered by disease or surgical intervention.

In this chapter, we discuss the methods of calculating corneal power, various instruments used to measure keratometry with their advantages and limitations, and corneal power estimation in challenging situations.

■ METHODS TO CALCULATE CORNEAL POWER

Corneal power or keratometry may be calculated using the principles of thin-lens paraxial formula, Gaussian optics, or ray tracing methods **(Table 1 and Flowchart 1)**. The keratometry readings obtained are not interchangeable, and the true net power and total corneal power measurements may not be used in conventional IOL power calculation formulas without conversion, as they are not calculated with the standard keratometric index of 1.3375.

Thin-lens Paraxial Formula

Conventional *simulated keratometry (Sim-K)* readings are obtained using the thin-lens paraxial formula.[2]

$$Power = (n1 - n0)/r$$

Where "n1" is the adjusted refractive index of 1.3375 based on the assumption of a constant ratio between the anterior and posterior corneal curvature, n0 is the refractive index of air (1) and r is the radius of curvature of the anterior corneal surface (in meters). The corneal power is based only on anterior corneal curvature measurements. Standard keratometric index of 1.3375 is used for calculation of sim-K, assuming a fixed posterior to anterior corneal curvature ratio of 0.822.

The keratometry readings are fairly reliable for virgin corneas; however, fallacious results are obtained in postrefractive surgery corneas, ectasia, or other conditions with altered anterior to posterior corneal curvature ratio.

TABLE 1: Corneal power measurements and calculation methods

Corneal power	Devices	Calculation method	Posterior corneal curvature measured	Refractive index used	Features
Sim-K	All keratometers, placido disk systems, optical biometers	Thin-lens paraxial formula	No	Standard keratometric index (n) of 1.3375—assumes fixed anterior to posterior corneal curvature ratio	Not suitable for cases with altered anterior to posterior corneal curvature ratio—postrefractive surgery, ectasia, etc.
True net power (TNP)/ Real Power (RP)	TNP—Pentacam (Oculus, Germany), RP—anterior segment OCT (CASIA 2, Tomey, Japan)	Gaussian optic thick-lens formula	Yes	Specific refractive indices of cornea (1.376) and aqueous humor (1.336)	Does not account for the spherical aberration of cornea (refractive effect)
Total keratometry (TK)	IOL Master 700	Gaussian optics thick lens formula	Yes	Specific refractive indices of cornea (1.376) and aqueous humor (1.336)	TK readings can be directly used with conventional IOL power calculation formulae and optimized IOL constants
Total corneal power (TCP)/total corneal refractive power (TCRP)/ mean pupil power (MPP)	Scheimpflug devices (TCP-Galilei, Ziemer; TCRP-Pentacam, Oculus; MPP-Sirius, CSO)	Ray tracing	Yes	Snell's law and specific refractive indices of cornea (1.376) and aqueous humor (1.336)	• Average 0.4–0.6 D lower than the simulated keratometry value • May not be used interchangeably with sim-K in current IOL power calculation formulas
Equivalent keratometry readings (EKR)	Scheimpflug devices (Pentacam)	Snell's Law	Yes	Snell's law and specific refractive indices of cornea (1.376) and aqueous humor (1.336)	EKR readings adjusted for those obtained using standard keratometric index of 1.3375—can be directly used with any two variable IOL power formulae. 4.5 mm zone EKR readings most accurate

(EKR: equivalent K readings; K: keratometry; Sim-K: simulated keratometry; SS-OCT: swept source optical coherence tomography; TCP: total corneal power; TCRP: total corneal refractive power; TNP: true net power)

Flowchart 1: Optical principles to calculate corneal power

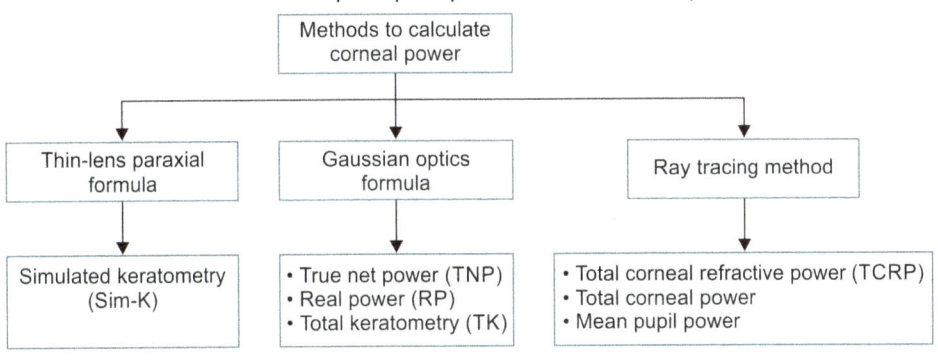

Thin lens formula is employed by manual and automated keratometers, placido disk-based topographers, and optical biometers to give sim-K readings.

Gaussian Optics Thick-lens Formula

Gaussian optics thick-lens formula may be used to assess the total keratometric power, which is referred to as the *True Net Power* (TNP) when obtained with Pentacam (Oculus, Germany), or *Real Power* (RP) when obtained with anterior segment OCT (CASIA 2, Tomey, Japan). Specific refractive indices of cornea (1.376) and aqueous humor (1.336) are used for calculation of the keratometry.

$$\text{Corneal power} = (n_1 - n_0)/r_1 + (n_2 - n_1)/r_2$$

Where n_0 is the refractive index of air (1), n_1 is the refractive index of the cornea (1.376), n_2 is the refractive index of the aqueous humor (1.336), and r_1 and r_2 are the anterior and posterior corneal curvature (in meters), respectively. A paraxial approximation is used for calculation, wherein the rays propagating through the posterior surface of the cornea are assumed to be parallel; this may lead to fallacious readings in cases with altered anterior to posterior corneal curvature such as postrefractive surgery. In addition, TNP or RP values may not be used directly in conventional IOL power calculation formulas.

Ray Tracing Method

Ray tracing methods use the *Snell's law* to calculate corneal power, taking into account the anterior and posterior corneal curvature, corneal thickness, and the actual refractive indices of cornea and aqueous humor.

Ray tracing technology is used to trace the incoming parallel rays through the anterior and posterior corneal surfaces. The actual refractive indices of air (1), cornea (1.376), and aqueous humor (1.336) are used to measure the focal length using Snell's law and convert it into the corneal power. Keratometric power assessed using the ray tracing method is referred to as the *Total Corneal Refractive Power (TCRP)* in Pentacam (Oculus, Germany), *Mean Pupil Power (MPP)* in Sirius (CSO, Italy), and *Total Corneal Power (TCP)* in Galilei (Ziemer, Switzerland). It is more accurate than sim-K values or TNP, especially in postrefractive surgery corneas. However, the ray-tracing keratometric values may not be used directly in conventional IOL power calculation formulae, as the formulae are optimized for corneal power values calculated using the standard keratometric index of 1.3375. The TCP measurements obtained by ray tracing method are 0.4–0.6 D lower than the simulated keratometry value.[3]

Equivalent K Readings

The equivalent keratometry readings (EKR) are obtained using Pentacam. Calculation is performed as per the Snell's law, taking into account the actual refractive indices of cornea and aqueous along with the anterior and posterior corneal curvature.

$$EKR = 0.376/r1 - 0.03165/r2$$

Where r1 and r2 are the anterior and posterior corneal curvature (in meters).

The keratometry values are adjusted such that they match the simulated keratometry readings obtained for a normal eye. Hence, EKR values may be directly used in IOL power calculation formulae that correct for the standard keratometric index of 1.3375.

Total Keratometry

Total keratometry (TK) values obtained using IOL Master 700 incorporate telecentric keratometry to measure the anterior corneal curvature and swept source OCT to calculate corneal thickness and posterior curvature.

A Gaussian optics thick-lens formula is used to give the TK values. The advantage of TK values obtained with IOL Master 700 is that it may be directly used in conventional IOL power calculation formulae with existing optimized IOL constants such as ULIB and IOLCon.org constants, without the need for additional conversion.

INSTRUMENTS TO MEASURE CORNEAL POWER

Corneal power may be measured using keratometers, placido disk-based topography devices, scanning-slit devices, Scheimpflug camera-based tomography devices, or optical coherence tomography-based devices **(Table 2 and Flowchart 2)**.

Keratometer

Keratometer is a device used to measure the anterior corneal curvature. It is based on the principle that the size of the image produced by the reflection of an object on the anterior corneal surface, which behaves as a convex mirror, varies with its curvature.

The corneal radius of curvature (R) may be calculated by using the formula "R = 2uI/O", where "u" is the distance of the image from the object, "I" is the image size, and "O" is the object size. Simulated keratometry or sim-K values are calculated based on the thin-lens formula using the anterior corneal curvature and standard keratometric index of 1.3375.

Keratometers may be manual or automated. The first manual keratometer devised by Hermann von Helmholtz used glass plates for doubling of the image and to displace the image by half of its length. The two images were aligned until their extremities touch one another; the total change in displacement gave the size of the image.[2] The position of the two mire images was adjusted by changing the position of the doubling device, while the mires remained stationary. The manual keratometers that were subsequently introduced include Javal–Schiøtz keratometer and Bausch and Lomb keratometer **(Table 3)**. They differ in the method of doubling and the method by which the mire images are aligned.

Ideally, no contact procedure should be performed prior to obtaining keratometry values. The keratometer should be properly calibrated and an average of at least 3 readings is used. In cases of any discrepancy in axis or K value, a repeat reading or a reading with another device should be obtained.

TABLE 2: Instruments to assess corneal curvature

Mode of keratometry	Measurement technique	Keratometry values obtained	Salient features
Devices measuring the anterior corneal surface:			
Manual/automated keratometry	Image produced by reflection of mires on cornea used to measure anterior corneal curvature	Curvature in the central 3–4 mm of the anterior cornea determined at two axes 90° apart	Provides the radii of curvature of the cornea, directions of the principle meridians of the eye, orientation and degree of keratometric astigmatism, and depicts presence of corneal distortion
Computerized placido disk videokeratoscopy	Corneal curvature measured based on the distance between rings formed by the reflection of concentric rings of a placido disk on the cornea	• Simulated K—simulates the traditional keratometry reading • Calculated as mean between the steeper and flatter corneal curvature values in 3–4 mm annular zone	• Estimates the corneal curvature and contour over 7–9 mm of cornea depicted as a color-coded map • Measure a larger range of corneal power than keratometers • Irregular astigmatism, corneal higher order aberrations, and corneal asphericity can be assessed
Optical biometers:			
IOLMaster 500	Measures the corneal curvature based on the relative positions of the 6 spots projected on to the cornea in a hexagonal pattern in 2.3 mm area (each spot is 1.3 mm from center)	The displayed steep and flat K represent the average keratometry values at two major perpendicular meridians	• Measures more central cornea than manual keratometers • IOLMaster uses telecentric keratometry • Lenstar LS 900 includes optional 11-ring placido disk topography module (T-cone) • Faster acquisition, less prone to motion artifacts
Lenstar LS 900	Measures 32 reflective light spots arranged in 2 rings, inner with 1.65 mm and outer with 2.30 mm diameter		
Devices measuring both anterior and posterior corneal surface:			
Combined slit scanning with placido disk topography	Placido disk and 40 slits sequentially projected on the cornea—anterior and	• Simulated K—Average corneal curvature over the central 3 mm derived from placido measurements	• Provides curvature, elevation and pachymetry map of the entire cornea

Contd...

Contd...

Mode of keratometry	Measurement technique	Keratometry values obtained	Salient features
(Orbscan II topographer)	posterior edges of the slits are analyzed to provide elevation and curvature maps	• Anterior, posterior, and total power maps—Derived from anterior and posterior curvatures of the cornea using slit scan measurements • Total optical power—Cornea's total effective power analyzed for the area of interest using Snell's law by ray tracing method	• Measures about 9,000 points over the corneal surface • Orbscan IIz incorporates corneal wavefront analysis
Scheimpflug imaging-based devices:			
Pentacam (Oculus Optikgeräte)	Computerized corneal topographer equipped with a digital Scheimpflug camera which rotates around the center of cornea	• Simulated keratometry—Obtained by averaging the sagittal corneal curvature (derived from anterior curvature) • True Net Power (TNP)—Sum of the anterior and posterior corneal powers calculated using Gaussian optical formula ($0.376/r_{anterior} - 0.04/r_{posterior}$) • Equivalent Keratometry Reading (EKR)—Adjusts corneal power using the formula ($0.376/r_{anterior} - 0.03165/r_{posterior}$) • Total Corneal Refractive Power (TCRP)—Derived using ray tracing calculation based on the anterior and posterior corneal radii and the pachymetry according to Snell's law	• Provides elevation, curvature, corneal thickness maps, and corneal wavefront analysis • Measures about 138,000 points over cornea • Can measure the central cornea as well, as the camera is not central • EKR readings unlike TNP and TCRP is adjusted such that it can directly be used in conventional IOL power formulae
Sirius Topographer (Costruzione Strumenti Oftalmici, Italy)	• Combined placido disk topography with Scheimpflug imaging	• Sim-K—Mean of the flattest and steepest meridian keratometric values obtained from average axial curvature from the 4th to 8th placido ring at each meridian	• Provides curvature, elevation, pachymetry map, and total corneal wavefront analysis of the entire cornea • Measures about 30,000 points over cornea

Contd...

Contd...

Mode of keratometry	Measurement technique	Keratometry values obtained	Salient features
	• Anterior corneal curvature data obtained from placido disk and Scheimpflug imaging. Posterior corneal curvature from Scheimpflug imaging	• True Net Power (TNP)—Calculated from the Gaussian optical formula using the anterior corneal curvature, the posterior corneal curvature, and the central corneal thickness • Mean Pupil Power (MPP)—Mean corneal power over the entrance pupil calculated by ray tracing through the anterior and posterior corneal surfaces using Snell's law	• Placido disk topography provides accurate data on anterior corneal curvature, surface irregularities, and tear-film quality
Galilei dual Scheimpflug analyzer (Zeimer)	• Combined placido disk topography with dual Scheimpflug imaging • Anterior corneal curvature data obtained from placido disk and Scheimpflug imaging. Posterior corneal curvature from Scheimpflug	• Sim-K—Average corneal curvature over the central 3 mm derived from anterior curvature measurements • Gaussian Equivalent Power—Calculated from the Gaussian optical formula using the anterior corneal curvature, the posterior corneal curvature, and the central corneal thickness • Total corneal power (TCP)—Average of corneal power for every detected point in a selected region of interest. Obtained using ray tracing of the anterior surface, posterior surface, and pachymetry data	• Provides curvature, elevation, pachymetry map, and total corneal wavefront analysis of the entire cornea • Measures about 122,000 points over the cornea • Placido disk topography provides accurate data on anterior corneal curvature, surface irregularities, and tear-film quality • Can reduce motion error by correcting eye motion and cyclotorsion
OCT-based device:			
IOL master 700	• Multidot keratometer projects the light onto the corneal surface at 3 zones (1.5 mm, 2.5 mm, and 3.5 mm) with 18 spots • SS-OCT used to compute posterior curvature from the corneal thickness	Standard keratometry (K)—Derived from the telecentric anterior corneal curvature along the 3 zones measured using reflectometry Total Keratometry (TK)—Combines the anterior curvature data with the posterior corneal surface, and corneal thickness	The TK values are adjusted to match the standard keratometry values, so it can be directly used in existing IOL power calculation formulae with the IOL constants

(IOL: intraocular lens; OCT: optical coherence tomography; sim-K: simulated keratometry)

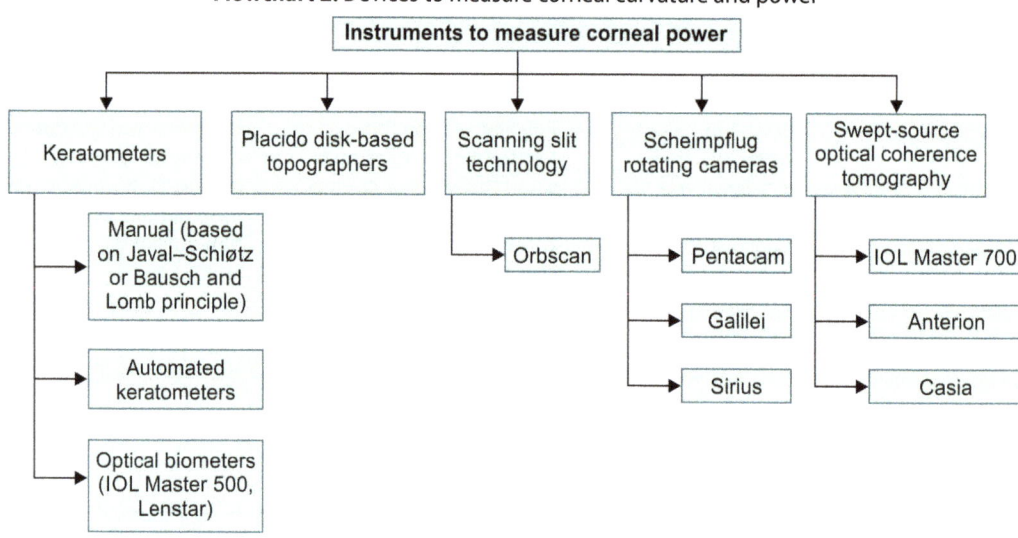

Flowchart 2: Devices to measure corneal curvature and power

TABLE 3: Manual keratometers				
Keratometer	**Doubling mechanism**	**Method to obtain reading**	**Variable features**	**Fixed features**
Javal and Schiotz keratometer	Wollaston prisms	*Two position keratometer:* Radius of curvature determined in one meridian-rotate optical system by 90° to determine radius of curvature in perpendicular meridian	Object size	Image size
Bausch and Lomb keratometer	Two prisms—one horizontal, one vertical	*One position keratometer:* Radius of curvature in perpendicular meridians determined simultaneously	Image size	Object size

- *Javal–Schiøtz keratometer:* The Javal–Schiøtz keratometer employs a Wollaston prism for doubling, incorporates a fixed doubling device while the mire separation is adjusted mechanically, and reading is obtained once they are aligned. The keratometry readings are taken along each meridian in two steps or positions.[4]
- *Bausch and Lomb keratometer:* In Bausch and Lomb keratometer, the doubling apparatus is variable while the object or mire size remains constant. It is a one-position keratometer wherein prisms are arranged simultaneously to produce doubling across the two principal meridians, such that readings from both can be taken once the mires align. The device has the advantages of easier visualization of the principal meridians and better ergonomics than the two-position instrument.[2]

- *Automated keratometers:* Automated keratometers follow the same basic principle as manual keratometers, except that the image reflected from the corneal surface is detected with a photodetector, which then measures its size and calculates the corneal curvature. Alignment can be performed simply by observing the mires on the display screen.[5] Handheld keratometers are also available wherein the operator assesses the correct instrument-to-patient distance from the pattern of reflected lights on the cornea. Automated keratometers are technically easier to use as well as less time consuming, and especially useful for examining children.[6]
- *Optical biometers:* Optical biometers such IOLMaster 500 (Carl Zeiss, Germany) and Lenstar LS 900 (Haag Streit AG, Switzerland) have an integrated automated keratometer for performing keratometry, and are discussed in detail in Chapter 4. Multiple light spots are projected on the cornea in 2–3 zones and the curvature is measured based on the relative position of these light spots on the corneal surface. The measurements are performed closer to the corneal center at the 1.6–2.3 mm zone. The biometers are less technician dependent with negligible inter-operator difference in measurement accuracy.[7]
- *Limitations:* Conventional keratometers measure the corneal curvature from 2–4 points at the 3–4 mm zone. The central or peripheral cornea is not assessed. Keratometry works on the theory of paraxial optics and is, therefore, unsuitable for measuring the peripheral cornea. Several assumptions are made while calculating the simulated keratometry. It assumes the cornea to be spherical or spherocylindrical in shape and symmetric, with major and minor axis separated by 90°. A standard keratometric index of 1.3375 is used, based on the assumption of a fixed anterior to posterior curvature ratio, which may not be accurate in postsurgical, ectatic, and scarred corneas with altered anterior to posterior curvature ratio.

  The accuracy is limited in measuring irregular, very steep or flat corneas. The range of keratometers is 36–52 D (6.5–9.38 mm), which may be extended to 30 D (5.6 mm), and 61 D (10.9 mm) by using a lens of –1.0 D and +1.25 D, respectively, in front of the keratometer's objective.
- *Sources of error:* Improper focusing of mires, faulty calibration, incorrect positioning of the patient, and excessive lid squeezing or lacrimation while obtaining the readings may lead to erroneous measurements. The user must adjust the focus of the keratometer for their own eye to avoid inducing measurement error.

Placido Disk-based Corneal Topography

Keratoscopy, like keratometry, measures the corneal radius of curvature by treating the corneal surface as a convex mirror.

It works on placido disk principle wherein a series of illuminated concentric rings is projected on to the anterior corneal surface to create a concentric ring image centered around the vertex. Corneal topographical assessment is performed based on the pattern and regularity of this image. The closer the mires, steeper the cornea. A much larger area of cornea is measured to provide a detailed assessment of its contour.[2]

Applications of placido disk topography have been further broadened by devices which employ computerized corneal mapping systems capable of processing information from thousands of points to produce detailed color-coded maps depicting the corneal curvature in a faster and more accurate manner. The instrument is aligned with the corneal vertex normal and measures 7–9 mm of the cornea. In addition to corneal power at various points, corneal topography enables detection of corneal shape abnormalities and evaluation of irregular astigmatism both qualitatively and quantitatively using the various topographic indices.[8] Modern topographers can also quantify the various types of corneal higher order aberrations including spherical aberrations which may help the surgeon to select an IOL with a specific asphericity that will best compensate for the patient's corneal spherical aberrations. In addition, observing the topographic pattern can alert the surgeon to the possibility of previous myopic or hyperopic corneal laser ablative procedures.[9]

Placido disk topographers have also been integrated in modern optical biometers such as Lenstar LS-900 (Haag Streit AG, Switzerland), Sirius Topographer (Costruzione Strumenti Oftalmici, Italy), and Galilei dual Scheimpflug system (Ziemer Ophthalmic Systems, Switzerland)

- *Limitations:* Like the keratometer, placido disk-based topography estimates the corneal power from the measured anterior corneal radii of curvature alone while assuming a constant ratio between anterior and posterior surfaces. Since the center of the placido mires is occupied by camera, the measured area is limited to the portion of the cornea (about 1.6 mm) that reflects the keratometric targets. Corneal power at the apex is extrapolated rather than measured.[10]

- *Sources of error:* The image attributed to corneal surface is in fact produced by the precorneal tear-film and may, therefore, be affected by tear-film irregularities such as dry spots or excessive tearing. In patients with dry eyes, applying a drop of lubricant before measurement may help obtain a more acceptable result. Fixation errors may arise if the patient is unable to concentrate on the fixation point due to large refractive error or low vision. Improper focusing of videokeratograph can affect the precision of readings. If too close to the cornea, the reading would be falsely high and vice versa.

Corneal Tomography

Corneal tomography represents a major advancement over placido disk-based topography and standard keratometry devices in being able to measure the posterior corneal curvature and corneal thickness in addition to anterior curvature. The measurement of posterior corneal curvature is of importance in cases where the normal relationship of both corneal surfaces are altered.[10]

Various modalities have been described for corneal tomography such as Scheimpflug imaging, slit-scanning tomography, and optical coherence tomography (OCT). The various systems employ different algorithms and formulae such as gaussian optics or ray tracing to calculate the TCP from the measured anterior and posterior corneal curvature. **Table 2** details the various devices and their measurement principles for estimating the corneal power. The significance of incorporating the posterior corneal curvature for estimating the corneal power has been discussed in detail in Chapter 5.

- *Limitations:* Corneal opacity or irregularity may obscure imaging of the posterior cornea and introduce artifacts into posterior corneal power calculations. Although the tomographic devices can measure both the anterior and posterior corneal curvature, each device uses a different formula to estimate the TCP from these measurements and is therefore not interchangeable. The discrepancy in the TCP values among different devices makes them unsuitable to be used directly in the existing IOL power calculation formulae and requires specifically calculated optimized IOL constants.

CORNEAL POWER MEASUREMENT IN SPECIAL CLINICAL SITUATIONS

Conventionally, IOL power calculation formulas use sim-K readings which may be obtained from any of the devices described in the earlier section. The assumption of a fixed anterior to posterior corneal curvature does not hold true in postsurgical and diseased corneas, and accurate corneal power measurements may be more challenging in these cases. **Table 4** summarizes the challenging clinical scenarios along with the preferred method of corneal power estimation.

Corneal Ectasia

Devices that measure corneal power based on anterior corneal curvature alone are bound to be inaccurate, with overestimation of keratometry values and subsequent IOL power underestimation. Scheimpflug imaging-based devices such as Pentacam (Oculus Optikgeräte) or Galilei Analyzer provide better repeatability of measurements. Total corneal refractive power (TCRP) or equivalent keratometry reading (EKR) from Pentacam has been associated with less hyperopic errors post-cataract surgery in corneal ectasia.[11]

Corneal Scars

The conventional keratometers that compute the corneal power in the 3-mm zone may give fallaciously high readings, as a paracentral region of steepening often surrounds the central scarred area. Moreover, keratometers may show irregular mires and fail to give reliable readings. Placido disk topography evaluates more corneal points and may compute the central anterior corneal curvature more accurately. Scheimpflug imaging provides further advantage over computerized topography in measuring the anterior corneal surface in highly irregular corneas, as the latter may fail to capture data over the abnormal surface due to incomplete mire registration.[12]

Endothelial Keratoplasty

In post-endothelial keratoplasty patients, the meniscus-shaped posterior lamellar graft in Descemet stripping endothelial keratoplasty (DSEK) or altered corneal posterior curvature after Descemet membrane endothelial keratoplasty (DMEK) contributes to the increased curvature of posterior surface resulting in a hyperopic shift. The use of keratometry measurements such as TCRP or $EKR_{4.5mm}$ that take into account both anterior and posterior corneal curvature may be more accurate for IOL power calculation.[13,14] In patients undergoing DMEK triple, IOL power calculation using pre-DMEK corneal power measured by ray-tracing or Scheimpflug tomography is less accurate, as the posterior corneal curvature is expected to change after surgery.[15] The use of pre-DMEK anterior corneal curvature, preferably measured using a Scheimpflug device, has been

TABLE 4: Corneal power measurement in special situations

Clinical scenarios	Source of error	Recommended technique for corneal power measurement
Post-radial keratotomy	• Keratometric index error—altered anterior–posterior corneal surface relationship • Radius or instrument error—optical center of cornea not measured by standard keratometers/topographers; measurements taken at 2–4 mm corresponding to steeper cornea • Formula error—Formulae using keratometry for ACD estimation results in an underestimation of ELP • Other sources of error—corneal irregularities, diurnal fluctuations in keratometry and the short-term and long-term hyperopic shift	• Use of more centrally measured corneal power using topography such as ACCP 3 mm of the TMS topographer in double-K formulae • IOLMaster standard keratometry reading used in Haigis formula
Post-myopic corneal laser ablative surgery	• Keratometric index error—altered anterior–posterior corneal surface relationship • Radius or instrument error—optical center of cornea not measured by standard keratometers and topographers • Formula error—formulae using keratometry for ACD estimation results in an underestimation of ELP in postmyopic laser refractive surgery patients	Standard keratometry values used in formulae such as Barrett True-K and Haigis-L provide very good outcomes
Post-endothelial keratoplasty	*Keratometric index error:* Increased posterior curvature due to shape of meniscus-shaped posterior lamellar graft after DSEK or altered corneal posterior curvature after DMEK contributes to the hyperopic shift	• Use of total corneal power estimates such as $EKR_{4.5mm}$ or TCRP preferred in post EK patients • Sim-K based on anterior curvature in patients undergoing simultaneous cataract surgery
Corneal ectasia	• Altered anterior–posterior corneal surface relationship—standard keratometric values overestimate the corneal power • Measured keratometry (K) may not equal that of the keratometry value at the visual axis as it may not coincide with steepest region • ELP error due to altered relation between corneal curvature and ACD • Reduced repeatability of readings due to corneal surface and tear film irregularities	• TCRP or equivalent keratometry reading (EKR) in cases with K<55D • Poor repeatability with all devices in cases with K>55D. Standard keratometry values (43.5D) preferable
Corneal scars	• Falsely high reading with conventional keratometers due to paracentral steepening surrounding the central scar • Unreliable readings with conventional keratometers due to irregular mires	Scheimpflug imaging or placido disk topography preferred for better measurement of central cornea and irregular surface

(ACCP: average central corneal power; ACD: anterior chamber depth; DMEK: Descemet membrane endothelial keratoplasty; DSEK: Descemet stripping endothelial keratoplasty; EK: endothelial keratoplasty; EKR: equivalent keratometry reading; ELP: effective lens position; K: keratometry sim-K: simulated keratometry; TCRP: total corneal refractive power)

recommended by some authors.[16] Adjusting the conventional keratometry according to the ratio of postoperative posterior corneal curvature and preoperative anterior corneal curvature has also been reported to produce more accurate refractive outcomes as compared to the use of conventional keratometry.[17]

Postrefractive Surgery

Standard keratometry measurements result in overestimation of corneal power after myopic laser ablative surgery. More recently, the use of total corneal power derived from direct measurement of posterior curvature has been performed; however, a significant percentage of refractive surprises are still reported. While the use of total keratometry in conventional non-LVC formulae might offer some benefit, the use of standard keratometry with newer formulae customized for post-LVC eyes such as Barrett True-K or Haigis L provides very good results.[18] Various methods of corneal power assessment and IOL power calculation in postrefractive surgery patients have been discussed in detail in Chapter 11.

CONCLUSION

Techniques of keratometry have evolved over the decades to provide more comprehensive and accurate measurement of the corneal shape and curvature. Most of the current IOL power calculation formulae are designed to use the corneal power derived from the anterior curvature. While this works well in virgin corneas, corneal power estimation using both anterior and posterior corneal surface measurements may be advantageous in toric IOL implantation or conditions where the assumption of normal physiological relationship of anterior and posterior corneal surfaces is no longer valid. Corneal power measurements obtained with different devices may differ due to differences in the corneal zone measured and the technology used, and should not be used interchangeably. With the myriad of modalities available today, a thorough understanding of the commonly used devices, their working principles, as well as how the different keratometry values are computed is crucial for optimal application of this parameter for accurate IOL power calculation.

REFERENCES

1. Zhang C, Dai G, Pazo EE, Xu L, Wu X, Zhang H, et al. Accuracy of intraocular lens calculation formulas in cataract patients with steep corneal curvature. PLoS One. 2020;15:e0241630.
2. Gutmark R, Guyton DL. Origins of the keratometer and its evolving role in ophthalmology. Surv Ophthalmol. 2010;55: 481-97.
3. Savini G, Barboni P, Carbonelli M, Hoffer KJ. Accuracy of corneal power measurements by a new Scheimpflug camera combined with Placido-disk corneal topography for intraocular lens power calculation in unoperated eyes. J Cataract Refract Surg. 2012;38:787-92.
4. Tennen DG, Keates RH, Montoya C. Comparison of three keratometry instruments. J Cataract Refract Surg. 1995;21: 407-8.
5. Nakada S, Tanaka M, Nakajima A. Comparison of automated and conventional keratometers. Am J Ophthalmol. 1984;97: 776-8.
6. Leyland M, Benjamin L. Clinical assessment of a hand-held automated keratometer in cataract surgery. Eye (Lond). 1997;11(Pt 6): 854-7.
7. Mehravaran S, Asgari S, Bigdeli S, Shahnazi A, Hashemi H. Keratometry with five different techniques: a study of device repeatability and inter-device agreement. Int Ophthalmol. 2014;34:869-75.
8. Wilson SE, Klyce SD. Advances in the analysis of corneal topography. Surv Ophthalmol. 1991;35:269-77.

9. Goto S, Maeda N. Corneal Topography for Intraocular Lens Selection in Refractive Cataract Surgery. Ophthalmology. 2021; 128:e142-52.
10. Holladay JT, Hill WE, Steinmueller A. Corneal power measurements using scheimpflug imaging in eyes with prior corneal refractive surgery. J Refract Surg. 2009;25:862-8.
11. Kamiya K, Kono Y, Takahashi M, Shoji N. Comparison of Simulated Keratometry and Total Refractive Power for Keratoconus According to the Stage of Amsler-Krumeich Classification. Sci Rep. 2018;8:12436.
12. Kanellopoulos AJ, Asimellis G. Clinical Correlation between Placido, Scheimpflug and LED Color Reflection Topographies in Imaging of a Scarred Cornea. Case Rep Ophthalmol. 2014;5:311-7.
13. Alnawaiseh M, Rosentreter A, Eter N, Zumhagen L. Changes in Corneal Refractive Power for Patients With Fuchs Endothelial Dystrophy After DMEK. Cornea. 2016;35:1073-7.
14. Xu K, Qi H, Peng R, Xiao G, Hong J, Hao Y, et al. Keratometric measurements and IOL calculations in pseudophakic post-DSAEK patients. BMC Ophthalmol. 2018;18:268.
15. Khan A, Rangu N, Murphy DA, Cooke DL, Siatkowski RL, Mittal A, et al. Standard vs total keratometry for intraocular lens power calculation in cataract surgery combined with DMEK. J Cataract Refract Surg. 2023;49: 239-45.
16. Debellemanière G, Ghazal W, Dubois M, Rampat R, Fabre L, Panthier C, et al. Descemet Membrane Endothelial Keratoplasty-Induced Refractive Shift and Descemet Membrane Endothelial Keratoplasty-Induced Intraocular Lens Calculation Error. Cornea. 2023;42:954-61.
17. Diener R, Treder M, Lauermann JL, Eter N, Alnawaiseh M. Optimizing intraocular lens power calculation using adjusted conventional keratometry for cataract surgery combined with Descemet membrane endothelial keratoplasty. Graefes Arch Clin Exp Ophthalmol. 2022;260:3087-93.
18. Sandoval HP, Serels C, Potvin R, Solomon KD. Cataract surgery after myopic laser in situ keratomileusis: objective analysis to determine best formula and keratometry to use. J Cataract Refract Surg. 2021;47: 465-70.

CHAPTER 4

Optical Biometry

INTRODUCTION

Precise biometry is imperative to obtain accurate results after cataract surgery. The advent of optical biometry at the turn of the century immensely improved the accuracy of ocular biometry and intraocular lens (IOL) power calculation.

Optical biometers allow single-step, precise assessment of axial length (AL) and keratometry as well as automated calculation of IOL power. IOLMaster (Carl Zeiss Meditec, Germany) was the first optical biometer introduced for commercial use in 1999, based on the principle of partial coherence interferometry (PCI). The following decade witnessed introduction of numerous other instruments essentially based on the same basic principle of time domain optical coherence tomography (TD-OCT), with some modifications and advancements. The next major step in this constantly evolving field has been the incorporation of swept source OCT (SS-OCT) in optical biometry, with enhanced speed and acquisition abilities.

In this chapter, we discuss the various optical biometers, their optical principle, measurements acquired, and formulae incorporated in various devices and clinical outcomes.

TYPES OF OPTICAL BIOMETERS

Optical biometers may be broadly classified into TD-OCT and Fourier Domain OCT (FD-OCT) based devices. In addition, combination devices that incorporate both corneal tomography and optical biometry have been introduced.

The TD-OCT-based devices include those using PCI [IOLMaster], optical low coherence reflectometry (OLCR) [Lenstar LS 900], and optical low coherence interferometry (OLCI) [Aladdin].

The FD-OCT devices include the newer biometers (IOLMaster 700, Argos, OA 2000, Eyestar 900, ANTERION) using the SS-OCT technology.

The AL scan (Nidek) uses PCI in combination with the Scheimpflug technology. In addition, two Scheimpflug camera-based tomographers have been redesigned to incorporate optical biometry function—the Galilei G6 (Zeimer) and Pentacam AXL (Oculus).

Table 1 details the measurement principles, illumination sources, and features of the different optical biometers. **Table 2** details the parameters measured by each device. **Table 3** describes the IOL power calculation formulae incorporated in the various optical biometers.

Partial Coherence Interferometry-based Optical Biometers

The IOL Master (Carl Zeiss Meditec, Germany) was the first commercially available optical biometer based on principle of dual beam PCI

TABLE 1: Types of optical biometers, measurement principles, and biometry parameters assessed

Principle	Device	Light source	Parameters measured and principle for each	Special features
Partial coherence interferometry	IOL Master 500	• PCI—780-nm MMLD • Illumination for WTW and Keratometry—880-nm LED • Fixation light for WTW, ACD and keratometry—590-nm LED	• AL: PCI • Km: Reflective keratometry at 2.3-mm diameter • Image analysis: ACD (with slit illumination), WTW	• AL reproducibility—0.025 mm • <60 seconds measurement time for both eyes • Dual mode—AL and Km acquired simultaneously • Telecentric keratometry • Marker less toric alignment
	Nidek-AL Scan	• PCI/LCI—830-nm IR diode laser • Scheimpflug imaging—470-nm LED monochromatic light • Keratometry—970-nm LED • Image analysis—525-nm LED	• AL: PCI/LCI • ACD, CCT: Rotating Scheimpflug imaging • Keratometry: Double-mire rings projected onto the cornea at the 2.4 mm and 3.3 mm zone • WTW, PD: Image analysis	• Repeatability of AL—0.017 mm • All parameters taken in a single step in 10 seconds • Automated 3D tracking • Optional built in ultrasonic biometer for AL measurement in eyes with dense cataracts • Markerless toric alignment
Optical low coherence reflectometry	Lenstar LS 900 (Haag-Streit)	• OLCR—820-nm SLD • Keratometry—950-nm LED	• AL, CCT, AD, ACD, LT: OLCR • Keratometry: Reflective keratometry with 2 rings of 16 light reflections each projected at 1.65 and 2.3 mm • WTW, PD: Image analysis	• AL repeatability—±0.035 mm • 3 seconds for measurement • 11 ring T-cone topography system up to the 6 mm zone • Assesses visual axis eccentricity • EyeSuite toric planner
Optical low coherence interferometry	Aladdin HW3.0 (Topcon)	• OLCI—830-nm SLD • Slit light projection for ACD—473-nm blue LED	• AL, LT, CCT: OLCI • ACD using reflection principle of horizontal slit light projection • Keratometry: From the reflection of 4 dedicated Placido rings at 2.4–3.4 mm • WTW: Image analysis • PD: Image analysis via IR and white LED	• AL repeatability—0.02 mm • Acquisition time—5 seconds • Keratoconus probability index • Zernicke Corneal WF analysis • 24 ring placido disk topography with a diameter of 8 mm • Dynamic, mesopic, and photopic PDs

Contd....

Contd...

Principle	Device	Light source	Parameters measured and principle for each	Special features
Fourier domain interferometry	IOLMaster 700	SS-OCT using 1055-nm tunable laser source	• AL, CCT, AD, ACD, LT, posterior corneal curvature: SS-OCT • K-Reflective telecentric keratometry using 3 LED rings at 1.5, 2.5, and 3.5 mm • WTW, PD: Image analysis	• AL repeatability: 8 microns • 2000A-scans/s • Both eyes measured in less than 45 seconds • Total keratometry (TK) measured • Full-length OCT image of eye showing anatomical details up to the fovea • Part of the Zeiss CALLISTO eye and Z Align system
	Argos (Movu)	• SS-OCT with 1,060 nm variable wavelength laser with 20 nm bandwidth • IR LED for keratometry	• AL, ACD, CCT, aqueous depth, LT, PD, CD: SS-OCT • Keratometry: Reflective keratometry with 16 IR LED source combined with OCT signals	• AL repeatability—10 microns • 3000 A-scans/s • Acquisition time less than 1 second • 2-D whole eye imaging based on SS-OCT • Enhanced retinal visualization for increasing sensitivity
	OA-2000 (Tomey)	OLCR using SS-OCT technology with 1,060 nm variable wavelength laser	• AL, ACD, LT, CCT: FD-OCT/OCLR • Keratometry measured at 2, 2.5, and 3-mm zones • PD, WTW: Image analysis	• AL accuracy: 0.03 mm • Scanning rate of 1,250 A scans per second • 3D eye tracking for B-scan imaging • Placido ring cone topography analyzes 9 mire rings projected on the cornea within a diameter of 5.5 mm • Automatic alignment and acquisition
	Eyestar 900 (Haag-Streit)	• SS-OCT biometry and imaging using 1,060-nm wavelength source (30 KHz scan speed) • Keratometry using 850-nm source	• AL, ACD, CCT, LT, topography (anterior + posterior): SS-OCT • Keratometry: Dual zone reflective keratometry measuring 32 points • WTW, PD: Image analysis	• AL repeatability—5 microns • Both eyes images in less than 40 seconds • Scan speed of 30 KHz • All parameters in a single measurement • B Scan imaging • Pachymetry map

Contd...

Contd...

Principle	Device	Light source	Parameters measured and principle for each	Special features
Combined tomographers with integrated biometers	Galilei G6 (Zeimer)	• OLCI—880-nm IR laser • Dual Scheimpflug imaging—470-nm blue LED • Placido disk topography—NIR 750-nm LED	• AL, ACD, CCT, LT-OLCI • WTW, PD: Image analysis • Posterior corneal curvature analysis using ray tracing: Scheimpflug technology • Placido disk topography using 20 rings	• AL repeatability = 0.025 mm • 60 images in 1 second • Total corneal WF analysis • Total corneal power and astigmatism • Iris based eye motion compensation • Pachymetric map • Corneal elevation data • Corneal ectasia screening
	Pentacam AXL (Oculus)	• Rotating Scheimpflug imaging—blue LED (475-nm UV free) • PCI	• AL: PCI • ACD, CCT, anterior and posterior corneal curvature: Scheimpflug imaging • WTW, PD	• Acquisition time—2 seconds • 100 images in 2 seconds • Zernike corneal WF analysis • TCRP, TNP • Holladay report with EKR • Topography, corneal elevation data • Ectasia screening • Meridional analysis using the TCP in 3-mm zone for toric IOL calculation
	Anterion (Heidelberg Engineering)	High-resolution SS-OCT imaging with a 1,300-nm source	• AL, ACD, CCT, corneal curvature (anterior + posterior), WF analysis: SS-OCT • WTW, PD	• Imaging app for visualization of AS SS-OCT images along with 3 optional Apps (Cornea, Cataract, and Metrics App) • Integrated ray tracing-based IOL power calculation (Okulix) • Total corneal power • Total corneal WF map • Spherical and toric IOL calculator

(ACD: anterior chamber depth; AD: aqueous depth; AL: axial length; CD: corneal diameter; LT: lens thickness; OLCI: optical low coherence interferometry; OLCR: optical low coherence reflectometry; PCI: partial coherence interferometry; PD: pupillary diameter; TNP: true net power; TCRP: total corneal refractive power; WTW: white-to-white)

TABLE 2: Biometric parameters measured by the various biometers

Optical biometer	AL	Km*	WTW	ACD	PD	LT	CCT	Corneal WF analysis	Placido disk topography	K_{Post}# or TCP
IOLMaster 500	✓	✓	✓	✓						
Aladdin	✓	✓	✓	✓	✓	✓	✓	✓	✓	
AL-Scan	✓	✓	✓	✓	✓		✓			
Lenstar LS 900	✓	✓	✓	✓	✓	✓	✓		✓ (optional T-cone)	
IOLMaster 700	✓	✓	✓	✓	✓	✓	✓			✓
OA 2000	✓	✓	✓	✓	✓	✓	✓		✓ (placido ring cone)	
Argos	✓	✓	✓	✓	✓	✓	✓			
Galilei G6	✓	✓	✓	✓	✓	✓	✓	✓	✓	✓
Pentacam AXL	✓	✓	✓	✓	✓		✓	✓		✓
Eyestar 900	✓	✓	✓	✓	✓	✓	✓	✓		✓
ANTERION	✓	✓	✓	✓	✓	✓	✓	✓		✓

*Anterior corneal curvature
#Posterior corneal curvature
(AL: axial length; ACD: anterior chamber depth; CCT: central corneal thickness; Km: keratometry; LT: lens thickness; PD: pupil diameter; WTW: white-to-white)

introduced in September 1999. It received the US Food and Drug Administration approval in March 2000. It used a Multimode Laser Diode (MMLD) infrared radiation of 780 nm of short coherence length (160 microns).[1,2]

Principle: A dual-beam version of partially coherent light beam is used to measure intraocular distances using interferometry. A superluminescent diode (SLD) is the source of light in present-day PCI optical biometers.[3] The light source with high spatial coherence and low temporal coherence is spilt using an external Michelson interferometer into a coaxial dual beam, with a temporal delay equaling twice the arm length difference, "d", of the interferometer. The dual beam illuminates the eye and each beam is reflected off both the cornea and retina. If the path difference, d, and the optical length (OL) are equal to each other (within the coherence length of source), the part of first beam reflected off the retina and the part of the second beam reflected off the cornea will overlap to create an interference pattern with fringes, or an interferogram. The presence of this interferogram detected by the photodetector confirms that the OL matches with d, and measuring the arm length difference of the interferometer shall give the OL measurement.[1,4] The optical length so obtained is divided by the composite group refractive index of the ocular media to obtain the geometrical AL. Dynamic assessment of interferogram fringes is based on the heterodyne detection principle, also referred to as Laser Doppler Interferometry.[1]

Parameters assessed: The optical biometer measures the AL along the visual axis, up to the retinal pigment epithelium (RPE).[1,5]

Axial length measured with PCI biometers is longer than those obtained using contact and immersion A-scan, as ultrasonic methods

TABLE 3: IOL power calculation formulae and aids incorporated in the different biometers

Optical biometer	SRK II	Haigis	Hoffer Q	SRK-T	Holladay 1	Holladay 2	Olsen	Barrett Universal II	Postrefractive surgery	Others
IOLMaster 500	✓	✓	✓	✓	✓	✓			CHM, CLM, Haigis-L	Phakic IOLs
Al-Scan	✓	✓	✓	✓	✓			✓ (optional)	Camellin-Calossi, Shammas-PL, Barrett True K (optional)	• SRK • Binkhorst
Aladdin	✓	✓	✓	✓	✓		✓	✓	Camellin-Calossi, Shammas no history Barrett True K	• Barrett toric calculator • Abulafia-Koch toric formula
Lenstar LS 900	✓	✓	✓	✓	✓		✓	✓	Barrett True K, Shammas No-History, Masket formulae	• Hill RBF • Barrett Toric calculator
IOLMaster 700		✓	✓	✓	✓	✓		✓	• Barrett True K • Haigis L	• Barrett TK universal, True K and Toric calculator • Haigis T
OA 2000		✓	✓	✓	✓				• Shammas PL • Double K SRK-T	• Showa • Haigis optimized • Okulix • Phaco Optics supported
Argos		✓	✓	✓	✓			✓	• Shammas no history formula • Barrett True K (optional)	Toric calculator
Galilei G6	✓	✓	✓	✓	✓				Shammas no history formula	Linked to Okulix ray tracing software
Pentacam AXL		✓	✓	✓	✓			✓	• Potvin-Shammas-Hill • Potvin-Hill (RK) Double-K formulas#	• Optional ray tracing software (Phaco Optics, Okulix)
Eyestar 900	✓	✓	✓	✓	✓		✓	✓	• Masket • Shammas no history • Barrett True K • Barrett True K Toric	• Hill-RBF • Hill-RBF/Abulafia-Koch for toric IOL • Olsen Toric
Anterion		✓		✓	✓			✓	• Barrett True K • Haigis L • Barrett True K Toric	Okulix interface Barrett toric Calculator

#Double-K Holladay 1, Hoffer Q, SRK/T
(CHM: clinical history method; CLM: contact lens method)

measure the AL along the anatomic axis till the internal limiting membrane (ILM).[5]

In addition to AL, the IOLMaster measures the corneal curvature, anterior chamber depth (ACD), and corneal diameter (CD) using image analysis, which may be used for IOL power calculation using the various built-in formulas incorporated into its software. ACD is calculated from distance between the corneal vertex (corneal epithelium) and the anterior surface of lens, calibrated against immersion ultrasound ACD results.

For keratometry measurement, 6 infrared (IR) diodes illuminate the cornea, the reflection of which is captured by a charged-couple device (CCD) camera and projected on the display. The instrument must be focused on the 6 peripheral dots arranged in a 2.3 mm diameter hexagonal pattern. The distance between the dots is used to deduce the corneal radius of curvature, and keratometric index of 1.3375 is used to convert the radius into dioptric power. To make the results comparable to that of other keratometers using a different keratometric index value, IOLMaster allows pre-selection of different index values.[6]

IOL power calculation formulae: Formulas incorporated in the device include Haigis, Holladay 1, Hoffer Q, SRK-T, SRK-II, and Haigis-L (in Version 4). Later versions allow computation of phakic IOL powers, additional AL measuring modes (silicone oil filled, phakic IOL in situ), and ability to acquire AL measurements even in dense posterior subcapsular cataract.

IOLMaster 500 (2010) incorporated telecentric keratometry or distance independent keratometry, wherein the distance between the spots remained constant irrespective of the distance between the eye and the device, allowing direct radius measurement.

Holladay 2 formula was additionally incorporated. It can also capture the reference limbal image as a part of Zeiss CALLISTO Eye and Z align for image-guided toric IOL alignment.

Optical Low Coherence Reflectometry-based Optical Biometers

The Lenstar LS 900 (Haag-Streit AG) is based on OLCR and was first introduced in 2008.

Principle: It uses a broad SLD source centered on a wavelength of 820 nm, coupled to a reflector. A standard Michelson interferometer is used where the optical length of the reference arm is changed using a rotating glass cube, which enables faster acquisition of A-Scans.[7] Lenstar captures 16 consecutive eye scans per measurement without the need for realignment, which are then superimposed to give a single composite A-scan.

Parameters assessed: Lenstar assesses the AL, keratometry (Km), white-to-white (WTW), central corneal thickness (CCT), ACD, and lens thickness (LT).

The AL, CCT, ACD, and LT are measured using OLCR. Dense Cataract Mode of measurement combines scans from all 5 measurements for evaluation to produce a composite scan in cases where individual reliable measurements could not be obtained.[8]

Keratometry and WTW are measured using image analysis. The aqueous depth is measured from corneal endothelium to anterior lens surface (internal ACD). This is then added to the CCT to acquire the ACD.[9] It also gives the retinal thickness (measured manually), pupil size, and eccentricity of visual axis from the corneal center.

An LED (950 nm wavelength) source measures corneal keratometry using 2 rings (dual zone keratometry) of 16 projected light spots each (total 32 spots) at 1.65 mm and 2.3 mm diameters. An effective refractive index is used to convert radius of curvature to the dioptric corneal power. All the above parameters are acquired in a single position without the need for realignment, thus shortening the examination time.

IOL power calculation formulae: The EyeSuite IOL is the IOL calculation tool suite on the Lenstar LS 900. In addition to the standard IOL calculation formulae like Haigis, Hoffer Q, SRK-T, SRK-II, and Holladay 1, it also includes the Hill-RBF method, Oslen, Barrett universal II formula along with the Barrett toric calculator. The LT measurement is advantageous when formulas requiring this parameter like Holladay 2 or Olsen (incorporated in the device) are used.[10] For postrefractive surgery patients, Barrett True K, Shammas No-History, and the Masket formulae have been included.

T-Cone Toric Platform provides true placido topography of the central 6 mm of the anterior cornea, and accurate keratometry readings at the 2.3- and 1.65-mm diameter optical zones. The device incorporates the EyeSuite Toric planner, an advanced toric calculator for precise planning of toric IOL implantation using high-resolution images.

The Lenstar uses a proprietary intelligent detection system that discontinues measurement in case the patient loses fixation and resumes measurement detecting correct fixation. The more recent Automated Positioning System (APS) uses dynamic eye tracking and allows the device to move autonomously during the automated measurement process. Other commercially available devices based on the principle of optical low coherence interferometry (OLCI) include the Galilei G6 (Zeimer) and Aladdin (Topcon).

Swept Source Optical Coherence Tomography-based Optical Biometers

The optical biometers based on SS-OCT technology include IOLMaster 700 (Zeiss), OA 2000 (Tomey), Argos (Movu), Eyestar 900 (Haag-Streit), and ANTERION (Heidelberg Engineering).

Principle: The SS-OCT is a type of Fourier Domain OCT where a tunable wavelength laser source rapidly scans through a series of wavelengths producing an interference pattern for each. A Fourier transform then decodes them into an A-scan, which can then be combined to form a B-scan. The advantages of SS technology include better penetration and faster speeds.[11]

- *IOLMaster 700:* IOLMaster 700 was the first SS-OCT-based optical biometer introduced in 2014, which uses a laser with a tunable wavelength centered on 1,055 nm. It provides a longitudinal section through the eye depicting the anatomical details of the ocular structures namely, cornea, AC, lens, vitreous, and the retina.

    Parameters assessed: The AL, CCT, ACD, anterior aqueous depth, and LT measurements are acquired using SS-OCT technology. A group refractive index is used to convert optical length to geometrical length and the measured AL simulates immersion ultrasound measurements using the built-in algorithm. The OCT uses 6 scan lines at 0, 30, 60, 90, 120, and 150° to measure the above parameters. The ACD is measured from the corneal epithelium to the anterior lens surface.

    The anterior corneal curvature measurements are acquired using telecentric keratometry wherein the device projects light onto the cornea at 3 zones namely 1.5 mm, 2.5 mm, and 3.5 mm (18 LED test marks). The posterior corneal curvature is measured directly using the SS-OCT technology to give the total keratometry or TK. The TK values may be directly used with the existing IOL constants on the User group for Laser Interference Biometry (ULIB).

White-to-white is measured using image analysis as in IOLMaster 500. A 1.0-mm horizontal OCT scan of the retina was also provided for confirming the presence of foveal pit in the captured scan, so as to ensure accurate fixation.[11]

IOL power calculation formulae: It includes a built-in Toric IOL power calculator, the Barrett Formula Suite (Barrett TK Toric, Barrett True K, Barrett Universal II, Barrett TK Universal II), and Haigis T (Haigis-Toric) formulas. Other useful features include a measurement caliper to visually confirm the displayed length of various parameters and the ability to detect macular pathologies while checking the fixation. The axial measurement of device enables a scan depth of 44 mm and tissue resolution of 22 microns.[11]

- *OA 2000 (Tomey, Nagoya, Japan):* It is an OLCR device based on swept source laser (1,060 nm) and placido disk topography for biometry. It is comparable to TD-OCT-based optical biometers in terms of the measurements obtained and refractive accuracy, but with a much better acquisition rate (98.5–100%) compared to them (64–95.3%).[12,13]
- *Argos (Movu, Nagoya, Japan):* It is a SS-OCT-based optical biometer that uses a 1,060-nm wavelength source with a bandwidth of 20 nm. Three OCT images are obtained for each measurement. The AL, ACD, CCT, aqueous depth, LT, pupillary diameter (PD), and corneal diameter (CD) are measured. The anterior corneal radius of curvature is derived from OCT in combination with a 2.1 mm diameter ring made up of 16 IR (860 nm wavelength) LEDs and is converted into the dioptric value using the keratometric index of 1.3375. The CD and PD are also measured using the data provided by the real time whole 2-D OCT image.[14]

The acquisition speed is faster with an A-scan acquisition rate of 3,000 A-scans/s. The internal algorithm uses a *segmental approach* for converting the optical distances into geometrical one, i.e., the individual refractive index from each segment namely the cornea (1.376), aqueous/vitreous (1.336), and the lens (1.410) is used and then summed up. Thus, it differs from other biometers (TD and SS-OCT based) which make use of a composite or group refractive index and assume that ratio between the length of the eye and its various components (such as lens, aqueous, vitreous) is constant.[15]

During acquisition, a camera provides a panoramic view of the eye, which allows for correcting the alignment of patient's eye in case of incorrect fixation. In cases of dense cataract, a software called "Enhanced Retinal Visualization" aids in measuring the AL accurately.

Corneal Tomography Devices with Incorporated Optical Biometers

The Galilei G6 and the Pentacam AXL are essentially Scheimpflug technology-based devices into which optical biometry function has been incorporated. Anterion is a swept source OCT-based device that enables corneal tomography, anterior segment imaging, and ocular biometry.

- *Pentacam AXL (Oculus):* The single rotating Scheimpflug camera device combines an additional module for optical biometry based on partial coherence interferometry (PCI), thus enabling assessment of anterior segment tomography, AL measurement, and IOL power calculation.[16]
- *Galilei G6 (Ziemer Ophthalmic Systems AG):* It is a new optical A-scan interferometer biometer that combines the functions of the Galilei G4, a placido-dual Scheimpflug tomographer with an optical A-scan device.[17]
- *ANTERION (Heidelberg Engineering):* It is a multimodal imaging platform based on the principle of swept source OCT images that enables comprehensive corneal topography and tomography, biometry measurements, and IOL calculation. It incorporates an Imaging app, Cornea app, Cataract app, and Metrics app. The Imaging app provides high resolution visualization of the entire anterior segment and the Cornea app allows detailed tomographical analysis. The Cataract app gives the ocular biometry parameters and incorporates several IOL power calculation formulae, including Okulix which is a new generation ray tracing-based IOL power calculation formula. The Metrics app enables measurements of angle parameters, anterior chamber depth and volume, lens thickness, and vault in cases with phakic IOL implantation.

OPTICAL BIOMETERS VERSUS CONVENTIONAL ULTRASONIC METHODS FOR AL ASSESSMENT

Axial length measurements obtained with PCI optical biometers correlate well with contact ultrasound biometry. PCI-based devices have better repeatability and higher precision than ultrasonic methods in both adult and pediatric eyes, as well as in extremes of AL.[18]

Most studies report higher AL with IOLMaster when compared to contact A-scan, with the difference ranging from 100 to 200 microns.[19] This systematic error may be attributed to factors such as corneal indentation during applanation, the difference in the retinal layer from where the measuring beam is reflected (ILM in ultrasonic methods vs. RPE in optical biometers) and difference in the measuring axis (visual axis with PCI vs. anatomic axis with ultrasonic methods).

The PCI-based devices have consistently shown more accurate or predictable refractive outcomes post-cataract surgery as compared to ultrasonic methods;[20] however, the difference became insignificant after A constant optimization.[21] Notably, a randomized controlled trial comparing ultrasonic methods and IOLMaster emphasized that the latter failed to acquire AL measurement in a significant proportion of patients, and that its superiority in terms of refractive outcome failed to persist when PCI failure eyes were not excluded from the analysis.[22]

Axial length obtained using immersion ultrasound is comparable to PCI-based optical biometers.[23] Optimization of the constant and taking into account the systematic error in AL measurement may further help improve the refractive outcomes when using immersion ultrasound.[24]

Advantages of Optical Biometers over Ultrasonic Methods

Optical biometers allow a noncontact procedure minimizing patient discomfort, eliminating the need for topical anesthesia, and reducing risk of epithelial abrasion or transmission of corneal infection. There are less inter-/intraobserver differences, more precise measurements, and shorter training times. Ultrasonic biometry is more time consuming compared to optical biometers, with latter often acquiring all the required parameters for IOL power calculation from a single device. The optical biometers have a better resolution; the IOLMaster has an axial resolution of 0.01 mm as compared to 0.2 mm with A-scan.[25,26] IOLMaster has both better accuracy and precision than ultrasonic biometry (0.02 mm vs. 0.1 mm). Immersion ultrasound has a precision of about 0.05 mm.

IOLMaster is free from errors caused by longitudinal eye movements, more reliable in myopic eyes and specially advantageous in challenging situations such as silicone oil-filled eyes, aphakic eyes, etc.

Disadvantages of Optical Biometers over Ultrasonic Biometry

An important limitation of time-domain OCT-based optical biometers is their inability to capture measurements in eyes with dense nuclear sclerosis or PSC. In PSC, the opacity is central and closer to nodal point therefore affecting a higher proportion of passing rays. Studies using earlier versions of IOLMaster reported a failure rate of 8–22%.[22,27] But this improved to about 3.7–4.7% with advances in the device software such as the addition of composite scan (IOLMaster version 5 onwards).[28] Similarly the Lenstar reported failure rate of up to 9–16%.[29] The failure rate reduced to <2% with system upgrades like the Dense Cataract Mode of measurement.[8]

Patients who are unable to fixate adequately due to inability to cooperate (e.g., children, mentally challenged), tremors, respiratory distress, severe tear film problems, nystagmus, lid abnormalities, and poor vision are poor candidates for performing optical biometry using TD-OCT-based devices, as the device depends on patient fixing on the laser light and measures along the visual axis.[2]

Visual axis opacities (e.g., keratopathy, corneal scarring, vitreous hemorrhage) may result in failure of scan acquisition. In addition, optical biometry cannot be performed in supine patients/intraoperatively or under general anesthesia.

COMPARATIVE EVALUATION OF DIFFERENT OPTICAL BIOMETERS

The biometric parameters obtained using the Lenstar LS 900 and IOLMaster have very good agreement with comparable repeatability and accuracy. AL measurements obtained by OLCR devices are slightly longer (0.01–0.02 mm) compared to PCI which may be attributed to the difference in respective algorithms used to recalibrate the optical biometry readings and improve their agreement with immersion USG readings. A meta-analysis by Huang et al. reported that all parameters (AL, ACD, and K) assessed using the two devices could be used interchangeably, except WTW which was lower with Lenstar.[30]

IOLMaster 700 has an excellent repeatability and reproducibility which is better than that of the PCI-based device.[11,31] The accuracy of IOL power calculation is comparable between the 2 devices; however, it is not recommended to use them interchangeably.

The success rate of IOLMaster 700 in acquiring measurements is significantly better than that of IOLMaster 500 and Lenstar, even in the presence of PSC, dense NS, or longer eyes (>30 mm). Failure rates of IOLMaster 700, Lenstar, and IOLMaster 500 in acquiring biometry measurements range from 0–4%, 0.7–28%, and 5–14.2%, respectively.[31-35] IOLMaster 700 is not as successful in acquiring scans in eyes with a total white cataract.[33,35]

Argos has excellent repeatability, with the measurements comparable to other biometers. Some studies observed smaller AL measurements compared to PCI or SSOCT biometers, with shorter AL measured in longer eyes and longer AL in shorter eyes, and comparable measurements in the intermediate AL range.[36] The use of separate individual refractive index to calculate the length of each segment may render the process of AL measurement more accurate in the shorter and longer AL eyes.[15] Similar to the IOLMaster700, Argos also has the advantage of a better acquisition rate, with the ability to capture scans even in the presence of advanced cataract. Its AL acquisition rate (96–98.2%) is better than PCI- and SS-OCT-based biometers.[14,36] Even in the subset of patients with advanced cataract (Grade 4 or higher), Argos could successfully acquire measurements in 89.9% of the eyes as compared to 63.6% by the IOLMaster 700.[37]

Scheimpflug-based devices with incorporated optical biometers, such as Pentacam and Galilei, have similar measurements and IOL power accuracy as compared with conventional PCI- and SS-OCT-based optical biometers, but with a wide range of differences in the variables assessed. Thus, the use of the measurements obtained using these devices interchangeably is not recommended.[38]

The A constants for the newer optical biometers using TD-OCT, swept source OCT, or Scheimpflug technology are usually adapted from the ULIB website, which are based on PCI measurements. It is suggested that surgeons perform constant optimization by personalization based on large-scale clinical data analysis for each device separately to achieve favorable results and accuracy in IOL power calculation.[9]

CONCLUSION

The technology in optical biometry continues to advance, with the newer SS-OCT-based devices featuring very high precision and faster speed of acquisition while allowing numerous parameters to be measured simultaneously. Technological advancements along with the incorporation of the newer advanced IOL calculation formula in the optical biometers have further improved the predictability and outcomes of cataract surgery.

REFERENCES

1. Hitzenberger CK. Optical measurement of the axial eye length by laser Doppler interferometry. Invest Ophthalmol Vis Sci. 1991;32:616-24.
2. Haigis W, Lege B, Miller N, Schneider B. Comparison of immersion ultrasound biometry and partial coherence interferometry for intraocular lens calculation according to Haigis. Graefes Arch Clin Exp Ophthalmol. 2000;238:765-73.
3. Hitzenberger CK, Baumgartner A, Drexler W, Fercher AF. Interferometric measurement of corneal thickness with micrometer precision. Am J Ophthalmol. 1994;118:468-76.
4. Fercher AF, Mengedoht K, Werner W. Eye-length measurement by interferometry with partially coherent light. Opt Lett. 1988;13:186-8.
5. Hitzenberger CK, Drexler W, Dolezal C, Skorpik F, Juchem M, Fercher AF, et al. Measurement of the axial length of cataract eyes by laser Doppler interferometry. Invest Ophthalmol Vis Sci. 1993;34:1886-93.
6. Vogel A, Dick HB, Krummenauer F. Reproducibility of optical biometry using partial coherence interferometry intraobserver and interobserver reliability. J Cataract Refract Surg. 2001;27:1961-8.

7. Schmid GF. Axial and peripheral eye length measured with optical low coherence reflectometry. J Biomed Opt. 2003;8:655-62.
8. Shammas HJ, Wetterwald N, Potvin R. New mode for measuring axial length with an optical low-coherence reflectometer in eyes with dense cataract. J Cataract Refract Surg. 2015;41:1365-9.
9. Hoffer KJ, Hoffmann PC, Savini G. Comparison of a new optical biometer using swept-source optical coherence tomography and a biometer using optical low-coherence reflectometry. J Cataract Refract Surg. 2016;42:1165-72.
10. Bjeloš Rončević M, Bušić M, Cima I, Kuzmanović Elabjer B, Bosnar D, Miletić D. Comparison of optical low-coherence reflectometry and applanation ultrasound biometry on intraocular lens power calculation. Graefes Arch Clin Exp Ophthalmol. 2011;249:69-75.
11. Bullimore MA, Slade S, Yoo P, Otani T. An Evaluation of the IOLMaster 700. Eye Contact Lens. 2019;45:117-23.
12. Reitblat O, Levy A, Kleinmann G, Assia EI. Accuracy of intraocular lens power calculation using three optical biometry measurement devices: the OA-2000, Lenstar-LS900 and IOLMaster-500. Eye (Lond). 2018;32:1244-52.
13. McAlinden C, Wang Q, Gao R, Zhao W, Yu A, Li Y, et al. Axial length measurement failure rates with biometers using swept-source optical coherence tomography compared to partial-coherence interferometry and optical low-coherence interferometry. Am J Ophthalmol. 2017;173:64-9.
14. Shammas HJ, Ortiz S, Shammas MC, Kim SH, Chong C. Biometry measurements using a new large-coherence-length swept-source optical coherence tomographer. J Cataract Refract Surg. 2016;42:50-61.
15. Goto S, Maeda N, Noda T, Ohnuma K, Iehisa I, Koh S, et al. Change in optical axial length after cataract surgery: segmental method versus composite method. J Cataract Refract Surg. 2020;46(5):710-5.
16. Sel S, Stange J, Kaiser D, Kiraly L. Repeatability and agreement of Scheimpflug-based and swept-source optical biometry measurements. Cont Lens Anterior Eye. 2017;40:318-22.
17. Ventura BV, Ventura MC, Wang L, Koch DD, Weikert MP. Comparison of biometry and intraocular lens power calculation performed by a new optical biometry device and a reference biometer. J Cataract Refract Surg. 2017;43:74-9.
18. Carkeet A, Saw SM, Gazzard G, Tang W, Tan DT. Repeatability of IOLMaster biometry in children. Optom Vis Sci. 2004;81:829-34.
19. Chia TMT, Nguyen MT, Jung HC. Comparison of optical biometry versus ultrasound biometry in cases with borderline signal-to-noise ratio. Clin Ophthalmol. 2018;12:1757-62.
20. Rajan MS, Keilhorn I, Bell JA. Partial coherence laser interferometry vs conventional ultrasound biometry in intraocular lens power calculations. Eye (Lond). 2002;16:552-6.
21. Bhatt AB, Schefler AC, Feuer WJ, Yoo SH, Murray TG. Comparison of predictions made by the intraocular lens master and ultrasound biometry. Arch Ophthalmol. 2008;126:929-33.
22. Raymond S, Favilla I, Santamaria L. Comparing ultrasound biometry with partial coherence interferometry for intraocular lens power calculations: a randomized study. Invest Ophthalmol Vis Sci. 2009;50:2547-52.
23. Whang W-J, Jung B-J, Oh T-H, Byun YS, Joo CK. Comparison of postoperative refractive outcomes: IOLMaster® versus immersion ultrasound. Ophthalmic Surg Lasers Imaging. 2012;43:496-9.
24. Kiss B, Findl O, Menapace R, Wirtitsch M, Petternel V, Drexler W, et al. Refractive outcome of cataract surgery using partial coherence interferometry and ultrasound biometry: clinical feasibility study of a commercial prototype II. J Cataract Refract Surg. 2002;28:230-4.
25. Packer M, Fine IH, Hoffman RS, Coffman PG, Brown LK. Immersion A-scan compared with partial coherence interferometry: outcomes analysis. J Cataract Refract Surg. 2002;28:239-42.

26. Eleftheriadis H. IOLMaster biometry: refractive results of 100 consecutive cases. Br J Ophthalmol. 2003;87:960-3.
27. Narváez J, Cherwek DH, Stulting RD, Waldron R, Zimmerman GJ, Wessels IF, et al. Comparing immersion ultrasound with partial coherence interferometry for intraocular lens power calculation. Ophthalmic Surg Lasers Imaging. 2008;39: 30-4.
28. Hirnschall N, Murphy S, Pimenides D, Maurino V, Findl O. Assessment of a new averaging algorithm to increase the sensitivity of axial eye length measurement with optical biometry in eyes with dense cataract. J Cataract Refract Surg. 2011;37:45-9.
29. Buckhurst PJ, Wolffsohn JS, Shah S, Naroo SA, Davies LN, Berrow EJ. A new optical low coherence reflectometry device for ocular biometry in cataract patients. Br J Ophthalmol. 2009;93:949-53.
30. Huang J, McAlinden C, Huang Y, Wen D, Savini G, Tu R, et al. Meta-analysis of optical low-coherence reflectometry versus partial coherence interferometry biometry. Sci Rep. 2017;7:43414.
31. Srivannaboon S, Chirapapaisan C, Chonpimai P, Loket S. Clinical comparison of a new swept-source optical coherence tomography-based optical biometer and a time-domain optical coherence tomography-based optical biometer. J Cataract Refract Surg. 2015;41:2224-32.
32. Kurian M, Negalur N, Das S, Puttaiah NK, Haria D, J TS, et al. Biometry with a new swept-source optical coherence tomography biometer: Repeatability and agreement with an optical low-coherence reflectometry device. J Cataract Refract Surg. 2016;42: 577-81.
33. Lee HK, Kim MK. Comparison of a new swept-source optical biometer with a partial coherence interferometry. BMC Ophthalmol. 2018;18:269.
34. El Chehab H, Agard E, Dot C. Comparison of two biometers: A swept-source optical coherence tomography and an optical low-coherence reflectometry biometer. Eur J Ophthalmol. 2019;29:547-54.
35. Hirnschall N, Varsits R, Doeller B, Findl O. Enhanced Penetration for Axial Length Measurement of Eyes with Dense Cataracts Using Swept Source Optical Coherence Tomography: A Consecutive Observational Study. Ophthalmol Ther. 2018;7:119-24.
36. Higashiyama T, Mori H, Nakajima F, Ohji M. Comparison of a new biometer using swept-source optical coherence tomography and a conventional biometer using partial coherence interferometry. PLoS One. 2018; 13:e0196401.
37. Tamaoki A, Kojima T, Hasegawa A, Yamamoto M, Kaga T, Tanaka K, et al. Clinical Evaluation of a New Swept-Source Optical Coherence Biometer That Uses Individual Refractive Indices to Measure Axial Length in Cataract Patients. Ophthalmic Res. 2019; 62:11-23.
38. Zhao J, Chen Z, Zhou Z, Ding L, Zhou X. Evaluation of the repeatability of the Lenstar and comparison with two other non-contact biometric devices in myopes. Clin Exp Optom. 2013;96:92-9.

CHAPTER 5

Posterior Corneal Curvature

■ INTRODUCTION

Estimation of corneal power and curvature is an essential component of intraocular lens (IOL) power calculation. Conventional keratometry techniques assess only the anterior corneal surface and are based on several assumptions, including a perfectly spherical cornea with a fixed anterior to posterior corneal curvature ratio, without taking into account the posterior corneal curvature or toricity. Posterior corneal surface also contributes to total astigmatism, which if not considered during IOL power calculation may lead to decreased accuracy and predictability of visual and refractive outcomes.[1]

In this chapter, we discuss the clinical significance of posterior corneal curvature and toricity, with methods to assess the magnitude of posterior corneal astigmatism and incorporate it in IOL power calculation (Table 1).

■ DEFINING POSTERIOR CORNEAL ASTIGMATISM

The anterior corneal surface acts as a convex lens. The toricity of the anterior cornea may be with the rule (WTR), against the rule (ATR) or oblique, and changes with age. The posterior corneal surface acts as a minus lens. It has an inherent toricity, with the vertical

TABLE 1: Characteristics of posterior corneal astigmatism

Magnitude	–0.3 D (range –0.26 D to 0.78 D)
Orientation	Against the rule
Age	Remains constant with age
Relation to anterior corneal surface	No significant correlation. Magnitude and axis may not be reliably predicted based on anterior corneal curvature assessment alone
Direct assessment	Devices based on Purkinje images (Cassini), slit-scanning (Orbscan), Scheimpflug technology (Pentacam, Galilei), swept source OCT (IOLMaster 700)
Indirect assessment	Nomograms (Baylor nomogram, Abulafia–Koch formula, etc.) and online calculators (Barrett toric calculator, Alcon toric calculator, etc.)
Clinical significance	Ignoring posterior corneal astigmatism leads to overcorrection of WTR astigmatism by 1.38×, undercorrection of ATR astigmatism by 0.65×

(ATR: against the rule; OCT: optical coherence tomography; WTR: with the rule)

meridian usually being steeper and resulting in ATR astigmatism. The posterior corneal astigmatism ranges from –0.26 to –0.78 D, with a mean value of –0.3 D.[2-7] It contributes to ATR astigmatism in nearly 80% of cases.[7]

CORRELATION BETWEEN ANTERIOR AND POSTERIOR CORNEAL ASTIGMATISM

There is no significant correlation between the anterior and posterior corneal curvature and astigmatism. Koch et al. analyzed the correlation between the posterior and anterior corneal astigmatism and observed a moderate correlation if WTR astigmatism is present in the anterior cornea, a poor correlation if oblique astigmatism is present in the anterior cornea, and no correlation if ATR astigmatism is present in the anterior cornea.[7]

AGE AND POSTERIOR CORNEAL ASTIGMATISM

The posterior corneal astigmatism remains constant with age and contributes to ATR astigmatism. This is in contrast to the anterior corneal astigmatism, which shifts from WTR to ATR astigmatism with increasing age. Koch et al. observed that 78.2% of their cases in their 20s had WTR astigmatism on the anterior corneal surface and only 6.9% had ATR astigmatism. In contrast, in their 80s, only 16.7% of cases had WTR astigmatism on the anterior corneal surface and 60.8% had ATR astigmatism.[7] Therefore, the posterior corneal astigmatism compensates for the anterior corneal astigmatism in the younger population and has an additive effect on total astigmatism in the older population.

MEASUREMENT OF POSTERIOR CORNEAL CURVATURE

Posterior corneal curvature may be measured directly using various topography and tomography devices. In addition, various nomograms and online calculators now employ corrective factors considering the posterior corneal astigmatism **(Flowchart 1)**. Ferreira et al. compared four methods of toric IOL power calculation—two methods that estimated the posterior corneal curvature (Barrett toric calculator and Abulafia-Koch formula) and two methods that directly measured the posterior corneal surface using the Scheimpflug imaging and ray-tracing software, respectively.[8] They observed that directly evaluating total corneal power for toric IOL calculation was not superior to indirectly estimating it using formulae and nomograms.[8]

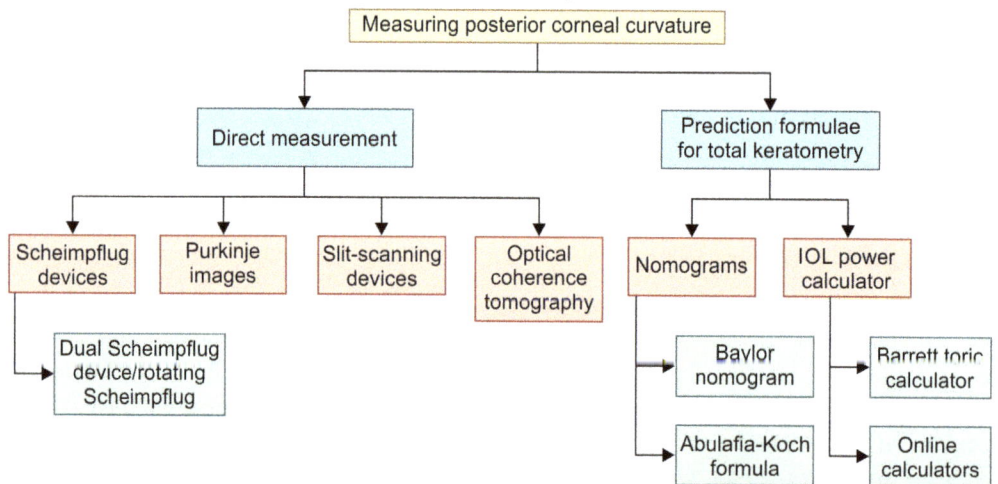

Flowchart 1: Methods for assessment of posterior corneal curvature

Direct Measurement of Posterior Corneal Curvature

Newer topography and tomography devices based on Purkinje images, slit-scanning technology, Scheimpflug technology, ray-tracing aberrometry, and optical coherence tomography allow a direct estimation of the posterior corneal curvature and provide total keratometry (TK) values taking into account both the anterior and the posterior corneal curvature **(Table 2)**.

IOLMaster 700 is based on the principle of swept source optical coherence tomography (SS-OCT) and combines three-zone telecentric keratometry with SS-OCT to provide TK values. TK values may be directly used with existing IOL power calculation formulae. In addition, the Barret TK Universal II (for nontoric) and Barrett TK toric formulae that use posterior corneal curvature measurements are directly incorporated into the device to provide accurate IOL power calculation.

Shammas et al. observed increased accuracy of astigmatic correction using the Barrett formula, when the keratometric values obtained from an OCT biometer were used in the formula as compared with using SimK values obtained using a Scheimpflug topographer.[9] Koch et al. observed that the Galilei Placido–dual Scheimpflug analyzer (Ziemer Ophthalmic Systems) had a lower predictive error in most eyes but significant prediction error of 0.57 D in eyes with WTR astigmatism.[10]

Hoffmann et al. compared five different systems for corneal power measurement

TABLE 2: Investigative modalities to assess preoperative keratometry

Instrument	Principle	Posterior corneal curvature	Technology
Manual keratometry	Doubling principle	No	Variable object size or variable image size using biprisms
Automated keratometry	Reflectometry	No	First Purkinje image used to calculate corneal curvature
IOLMaster 700	Partial coherence interferometry	Yes	Integrated swept source OCT technology with retinal OCT scan
Lenstar LS 900®	Optical low-coherence reflectometry	No Incorporates Barrett	Double-ring Placido disk topographer, integrated EyeSuite toric software with Hill RBF, Barrett, and Olsen formula
Orbscan IIz	Placido disc and slit scanning topography	Yes	Digitally recreates posterior corneal curvature using triangulation of the previously generated elevation and anterior topography
Pentacam	Scheimpflug imaging	Yes	Compensates for ocular movements
Galilei	Ray-tracing technology	Yes	Uses revolving dual-channel Scheimpflug camera with Placido disc technology
Cassini corneal shape analyzer	LED ray-tracing technology	Yes	Uses color diode lights 2nd Purkinje imaging technology for posterior cornea
Anterion	Swept source OCT	Yes	High-resolution SS-OCT imaging with a 1,300-nm source. Integrated ray tracing-based IOL power calculation (Okulix)

(IOL: intraocular lens; LED: light-emitting diode; OCT: optical coherence tomography; RBF: radial basis function)

including a swept source Fourier domain OCT, an autokeratometer, a hybrid topographer, a Placido topographer, and a Scheimpflug tomographer. They observed more precise results with OCT and hybrid topography systems that incorporate posterior curvature measurements.[11] Scheimpflug-based systems directly measure the posterior corneal curvature; however, they have the disadvantage of high measuring noise. The highest precision for planning toric IOL power and axis was achieved by combining the keratometry and OCT data.

Prediction Formulae for Total Keratometry

Baylor nomogram and Abulafia-Koch formula incorporate corrective factors for posterior corneal astigmatism. In addition, online calculators are available, including Barrett online calculator and various toric calculators, that take into account TK values.

Baylor nomogram aims to leave patients with slight WTR astigmatism to account for the ATR shift that occurs over time with aging **(Table 3)**.[10] It takes into account the surgically induced astigmatism as well. In cases with WTR astigmatism, Baylor's nomogram shifts the threshold for selecting a toric IOL up 0.7 D, so that a toric IOL is not used until the anterior cornea has 1.7 D of WTR astigmatism. In cases with ATR astigmatism, the nomogram shifts the threshold for selecting a toric IOL down 0.7 D, so that in an eye with 0.8 D of ATR astigmatism, a toric IOL of 1.5 D of toricity is used. It has been observed to be more precise than Alcon and Holladay toric calculators.

Abulafia-Koch formula is a regression formula that calculates estimated total corneal astigmatism based on standard keratometry measurements.[12] It has similar outcomes to Barrett toric calculator.

Barett toric calculator takes into account both effective lens position (ELP) and posterior corneal astigmatism **(Fig. 1)**. It has better predictability than the Baylor nomogram and Holladay and Alcon toric calculators. Online calculators have been revised to incorporate corrections for posterior corneal curvature. Revised AcrySof toric calculator incorporates the Barret toric algorithm **(Fig. 2)** and the Tecnis calculator incorporates posterior corneal astigmatism compensation.

■ CLINICAL SIGNIFICANCE

Estimation of posterior corneal astigmatism assumes significance in cases planned for premium IOL implantation, such as toric and multifocal IOLs.[13] When implanting a toric IOL, relying on anterior corneal astigmatism alone leads to an overcorrection of WTR astigmatism by a factor of 1.38 and an undercorrection of ATR astigmatism by a factor of 0.65.[14]

The threshold for implantation of toric multifocal IOLs is lower than toric monofocal IOLs, as residual astigmatism is not well tolerated in cases with multifocal IOLs and results in suboptimal patient satisfaction. TK estimation is essential in these cases, as illustrated in the case example **(Fig. 3)**.

TABLE 3: Baylor toric IOL nomogram

Effective IOL cylinder power at corneal plane (D)	WTR (D)	ATR (D)
0.00	≤1.69 (PCRI if >1.00)	<0.39
1.00	1.70–2.19	0.40–0.79
1.50	2.20–2.69	0.80–1.29
2.00	2.70–3.19	1.30–1.79
2.50	3.20–3.79	1.80–2.29
3.00	3.80–4.39	2.30–2.79
3.50	4.40–4.99	2.80–3.29
4.00	5.00	3.30–3.79

Note: Values in the table are the vector sum of the anterior corneal and surgically induced astigmatism. (ATR: against the rule; IOL: intraocular lens; PCRI: peripheral corneal relaxing incision; WTR: with the rule)

CHAPTER 5: Posterior Corneal Curvature

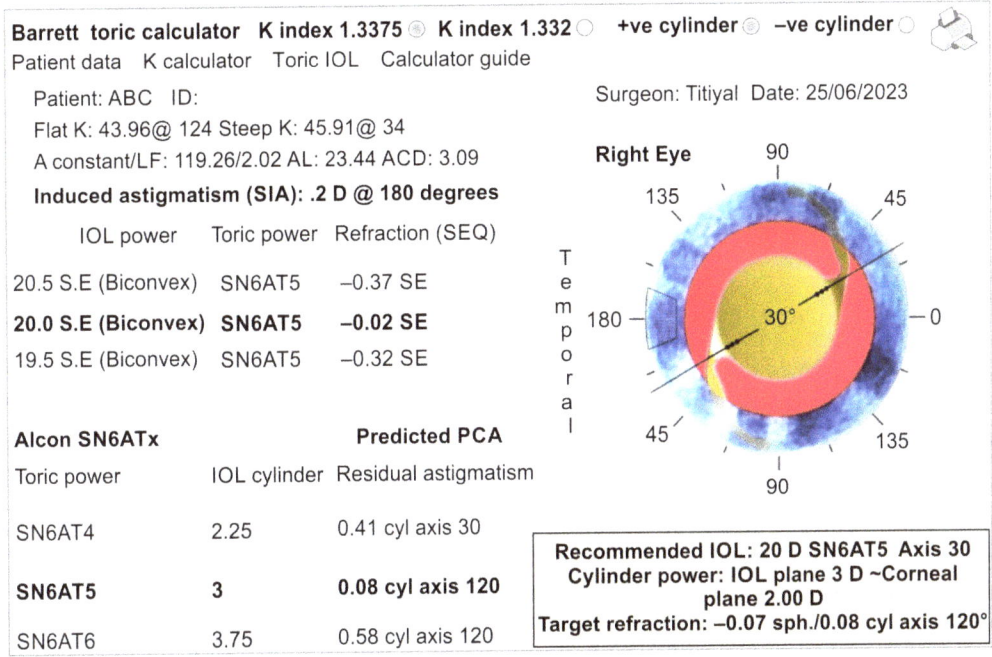

Fig. 1: Barrett online toric calculator

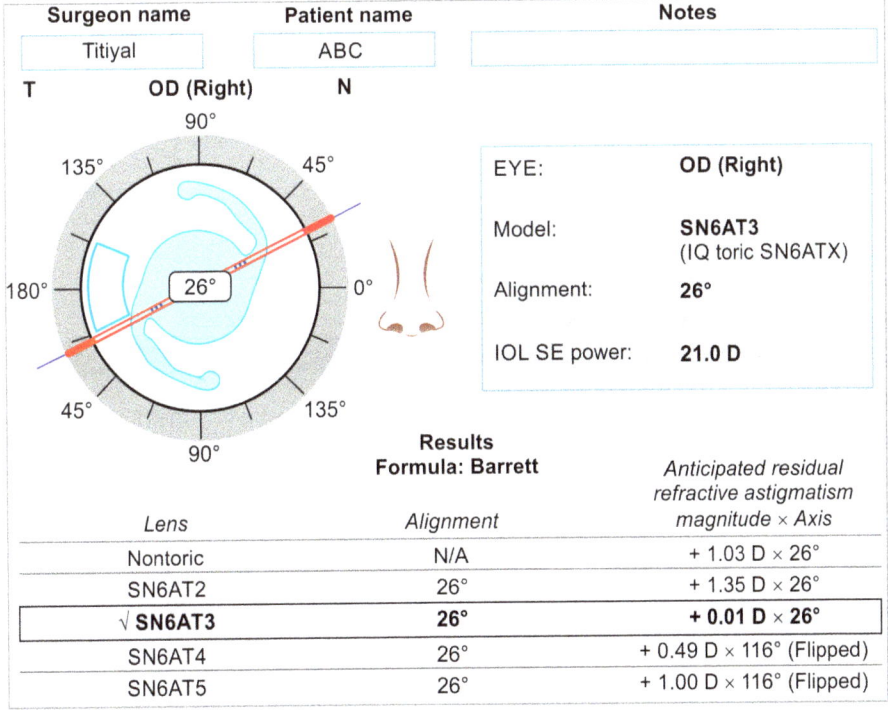

Fig. 2: Alcon online toric calculator incorporates Barrett calculator (Medical Chart)

Toric SN6AT(2–9) - Barrett TK Toric - T3				
Eye status				
LS: Phakic Ref: — LVC: Untreated Target ref: –0.20 D			VS: Vitreous body VA — LVC mode: – SIA: +0.10 D @ 180°	
Metric values				
AL: 23.66 mm		SD: 13 µm		
ACD: 3.09 mm		SD: 8 µm		
LT: 4.10 mm		SD: 12 µm		
WTW: 11.6 mm				
SE: 44.56 D		SD: 0.01 D	K1: 44.19 D	@ 52°
ΔK : +0.74 D		@142°	K2: 44.93 D	@ 142°
TSE: 44.59 D		SD: 0.04D	TK1: 44.15 D	@ 65°
ΔTK: +0.89D		@155°	TK2: 45.04 D	@ 155°

TK Alcon SN60WF IQ (India)
–Barrett TK universal II–
LF: +1.83 DF: +5.0

IOL (D)	Ref (D)
+20.50	–0.94
+20.00	–0.58
+19.50	**–0.22**
+19.00	+0.13
+18.50	+0.48
+19.19	Emmetropia

TK AMO Tecnis Eyhance
–Barrett TK universal II–
LF: +2.09 DF: +4.0

IOL (D)	Ref (D)
+21.00	–0.94
+20.50	–0.59
+20.00	**–0.24**
+19.50	+0.10
+19.00	+0.44
+19.66	Emmetropia

TK Alcon toric SN6AT (2–9)
–Barrett TK Toric–
LF: +2.02 DF: +5.0

IOL SE	IOL Cyl	IOL axis	Ref SE	Ref Sph	Ref Cyl	Ref Axis
T2 +21.00	+1.00	157°	–1.04	–1.13	+0.19	157°
T2 +20.50	+1.00	157°	–0.68	–0.78	+0.19	157°
T2 +20.00	**+1.00**	**157°**	**–0.33**	**–0.43**	**+0.19**	**157°**
T2 +19.50	+1.00	157°	+0.02	–0.08	+0.19	157°
T2 +19.00	+1.00	157°	+0.36	+0.26	+0.19	157°
+19.50	+1.25	157°	Emmetropia			
T3 +20.00	+1.50	157°	–0.33	–0.40	+0.14	67°

Fig. 3: Case example demonstrating significance of posterior corneal astigmatism in IOL power calculation for premium IOL. A 45-year-old female presented with posterior subcapsular cataract in left eye and was planned for multifocal IOL implantation. The astigmatism based on SimK values taking into account only the anterior corneal surface was 0.74 D (red box). However, astigmatism taking into account TK including the posterior corneal astigmatism was 0.89 D (green box). Based on the TK values, the patient was planned for a multifocal toric IOL, rather than plain multifocal IOL. Implanting a plain multifocal IOL in this case based on SimK values would have resulted in residual postoperative cylinder with suboptimal visual outcomes

The ratio of the anterior to the posterior corneal curvature is also altered after cornea-based refractive surgical procedures, including photorefractive keratectomy (PRK), laser-assisted in situ keratomileusis (LASIK), and radial keratotomy. Similarly, corneal ectatic disorders also require accurate assessment of both anterior and posterior corneal curvature and astigmatism for accurate calculations.

■ CONCLUSION

Conventional keratometry estimation techniques were based on anterior corneal surface measurements alone and did not take into account the toricity of the posterior corneal surface. Posterior corneal surface also contributes to total corneal astigmatism, with a magnitude of –0.3 D, that is ATR, and remains constant with age. There is no significant correlation between anterior and posterior corneal surfaces, and posterior corneal astigmatism may not be predicted based on anterior corneal curvature assessment. Ignoring posterior corneal astigmatism will lead to decreased accuracy of IOL power calculation, especially in cases planned for premium IOLs including toric and multifocal IOLs. The newer topography and tomography devices enable direct measurement of the posterior corneal surface. In addition, various nomograms and online calculators employ correction factors to account for posterior corneal astigmatism. Direct measurement of posterior corneal curvature is not superior to estimating it using formulae and nomograms; however, it is essential to account for posterior corneal astigmatism for enhanced refractive accuracy.

■ REFERENCES

1. Ho J-D, Tsai C-Y, Liou S-W. Accuracy of corneal astigmatism estimation by neglecting the posterior corneal surface measurement. Am J Ophthalmol. 2009;147:788-95.
2. Royston JM, Dunne MCM, Barnes DA. Measurement of posterior corneal surface Toricity. Optom Vis Sci. 1990;67:757.
3. Dunne MC, Royston JM, Barnes DA. Posterior corneal surface toricity and total corneal astigmatism. Optom Vis Sci Off Publ Am Acad Optom. 1991;68:708-10.
4. Dubbelman M, Sicam VADP, Van der Heijde GL. The shape of the anterior and posterior surface of the aging human cornea. Vision Res. 2006;46:993-1001.
5. Prisant O, Hoang-Xuan T, Proano C, Hernandez E, Awwad ST, Azar DT. Vector summation of anterior and posterior corneal topographical astigmatism. J Cataract Refract Surg. 2002;28:1636-43.
6. Módis L, Langenbucher A, Seitz B. Evaluation of normal corneas using the scanning-slit topography/pachymetry system. Cornea. 2004;23:689-94.
7. Koch DD, Ali SF, Weikert MP, Shirayama M, Jenkins R, Wang L. Contribution of posterior corneal astigmatism to total corneal astigmatism. J Cataract Refract Surg. 2012;38: 2080-7.
8. Ferreira TB, Ribeiro P, Ribeiro FJ, O'Neill JG. Comparison of methodologies using estimated or measured values of total corneal astigmatism for toric intraocular lens power calculation. J Refract Surg. 2017;33:794-800.
9. Shammas HJ, Yu F, Shammas MC, Jivrajka R, Hakimeh C. Predicted vs measured posterior corneal astigmatism for toric intraocular lens calculations. J Cataract Refract Surg. 2022; 48:690-6.
10. Koch DD, Jenkins RB, Weikert MP, Yeu E, Wang L. Correcting astigmatism with toric intraocular lenses: effect of posterior corneal astigmatism. J Cataract Refract Surg. 2013;39: 1803-9.
11. Hoffmann PC, Abraham M, Hirnschall N, Findl O. Prediction of residual astigmatism after cataract surgery using swept source Fourier domain optical coherence tomography. Curr Eye Res. 2014;39:1178-86.
12. Abulafia A, Koch DD, Wang L, Hill WE, Assia EI, Franchina M, et al. New regression formula for toric intraocular lens calculations. J Cataract Refract Surg. 2016;42:663-71.
13. Mohammadi S-F, Khorrami-Nejad M, Hamidirad M. Posterior corneal astigmatism: A review article. Clin Optom. 2019;11:85-96.
14. Goggin M, Zamora-Alejo K, Esterman A, van Zyl L. Adjustment of anterior corneal astigmatism values to incorporate the likely effect of posterior corneal curvature for toric intraocular lens calculation. J Refract Surg. 2015;31:98-102.

SECTION 3

Intraocular Lens Power Calculation Formulae

6. Regression Formulae
7. Vergence Formulae
8. Aberrometry-based Formulae
9. Artificial Intelligence in Intraocular Lens Power Calculation

CHAPTER 6

Regression Formulae

■ INTRODUCTION

Intraocular lens (IOL) power calculation formulae have continued to evolve since the introduction of the first theoretical formula by Fyodorov in 1967. Theoretical formulae were derived from mathematical considerations based on the optics of eye. Regression formulae marked the next major advance in IOL power calculation formulae and are empirically derived from the linear regression analysis of a large number of eyes that have undergone IOL implantation.

The first regression formula, Sanders-Retzlaff-Kraff (SRK) formula, was introduced in 1980.[1,2] Other regression formulae including Gills formula, Axt formula, and Donzis-Kastle-Gordon (DKG) formula were subsequently introduced but did not gain as much popularity.[3] Subsequent generations of IOL power formulae, which provided a better estimation of effective lens position using vergence, artificial intelligence, and ray-tracing approaches, have since replaced regression formulae.

With the advent of optical biometry, easy access to various online calculators, and newer generation formulae, the role of regression formulae is extremely limited. However, many of the newer formulae include some element of regression in them, underscoring the importance of understanding the basic principle, advantages, and shortcomings.

■ PRINCIPLE

Regression analysis is a method for deriving an equation to fit an assumed relationship between two variables. Empirical formulae employ regression analysis on retrospective data from a large series of eyes that underwent IOL implantation to derive a formula evaluating the relationship between axial length (AL), keratometry, and IOL power to be implanted. They essentially use a statistical approach to generate a mean value and incorporate a regression coefficient for correction of deviations from this mean value.[2,4]

■ SANDERS–RETZLAFF–KRAFF (SRK) FORMULA

The authors Sanders, Kraff, and Retzlaff studied a series of eyes that underwent cataract surgery with IOL implantation using regression analysis to derive a new formula that predicted the required IOL power.[1,2,5]

$$\text{Predicted IOL power} = A + 2.5 \, (AL) + 0.9 \, (\text{keratometry})$$

where the value of constant "A" differed based on each type of lens implant and manufacturer.

Unlike the older theoretical formulae, the authors concluded that the IOL power accuracy depended primarily on AL and corneal dioptric power rather than the postoperative anterior chamber depth (ACD) and refractive indices of aqueous and vitreous. The SRK formula was found to be superior in accuracy to the theoretical formulae while incorporating fewer variables.[2]

SRK II Formula

The accuracy of SRK formula was restricted to average eyes with an AL ranging from 22.0 to 24.5 mm. A lower IOL power was predicted for smaller eyes (<22 mm) and a higher power was predicted for longer eyes (>24.5 mm). The SRK II formula aimed to improve the accuracy of IOL power calculation in the long and shorter eyes by taking into account the nonlinear relationship between AL and IOL power. A simplified stepwise approximation was used to incorporate a correction factor in the original SRK formula to increase the IOL power in shorter eyes and decrease it in longer eyes **(Table 1)**.[6] The formula allows the surgeons to simply add or subtract the correction factor from the calculated SRK predictions without the need of any sophisticated calculations.

The authors also provided a formula which helped determine the IOL power to be implanted (I) to produce a given postoperative refractive error (R):

$$I = P - (R \times CR)$$

where P = IOL power calculated with SRK II formula for emmetropia, and CR = 1, if P ≤ 14; CR = 1.25, if P > 14.

MODIFICATIONS OF SRK FORMULA

Dang and Raj suggested modifications of the A constant used in the SRK II formula to make it surgeon-specific and enhance its predictive accuracy **(Table 2)**. The modifications led to 80% of eyes having a residual refractive error of <1 D.[7]

The SRK formula tends to overcorrect in cases with longer AL with resultant postoperative myopic residual error. Kora et al. suggested further modification of SRK formula to improve its predictability in severely myopic eyes with long AL.[8] As per their modification, the L-SRK formula for long eyes is calculated as

$$I = A - 2.5L - 0.9K - 1.69R - 1.69$$

where I is the actual implanted IOL power, A is the A constant, L is the AL, K is the mean keratometry, and R is the predicted postoperative refraction. Kora et al. also suggested further modification of SRK formula for AL between 24.5 and 27.0 mm to decrease the incidence of postoperative myopia.[9]

TABLE 1: The modified A constant for SRK II formula based on the axial length

Axial length	A1 (modified A constant)
AL <20 mm	A + 3
20 mm ≤AL <21 mm	A + 2
21 mm ≤AL <22 mm	A + 1
22 mm ≤AL <24.5 mm	A
AL ≥24.5 mm	A − 0.5

(A: constant from the original SRK formula; AL: axial length; SRK II: Sanders–Retzlaff–Kraff II)

TABLE 2: Surgeon-specific SRK II formula

Axial length	A1 (modified A constant)
AL <20 mm	A1 = A + 1.5
AL ≥20 mm and <21 mm	A1 = A + 1.0
AL ≥21 mm and >22 mm	A1 = A + 0.5
AL ≥22 mm and <24.5 mm	A
AL ≥24.5 mm and <26.0 mm	A1 = A − 1.0
AL >26.0 mm	A1 = A − 1.5

(A: constant from the original SRK formula; AL: axial length; SRK II: Sanders–Retzlaff–Kraff II)
Source: Dang and Raj (1989).

OUTCOMES WITH REGRESSION FORMULAE

SRK formula demonstrated a better accuracy as compared to the older theoretical formulae with 63–79% of eyes achieving errors of <1 D.[2,10] With the use of SRK II formula, Sanders et al. reported 80% and 30% eyes within errors of <1 D and <0.5 D, respectively. Among the short eyes (<22 mm), 74.0% were corrected to within 1 D with SRK II as opposed to 63% with SRK; among long eyes (≥24.5 mm), 78.0% of cases demonstrated <1.0 D error with SRK II as compared to 65% with SRK formula.[6,7] Third-generation IOL power calculation formulae including the SRK theoretical (SRK-T), Hoffer Q, and Holladay 1 formula superseded the SRK II formula in terms of prediction accuracy, particularly in the long and short eyes.[11,12] Sanders et al. reported a poor accuracy with SRK II formula in extremely long eyes (AL > 28.4 mm), with only 28% eyes achieving a <1 D prediction error.[13]

LIMITATIONS OF REGRESSION FORMULAE

The accuracy of regression formulae depends on the data set from which it is derived. Inhomogeneity in patient data due to differences in surgical technique or biometric measurements can affect the accuracy of formulae. A change in the technique of biometry or IOL position may change the regression coefficients.[4] The regression formulae are much less accurate in extreme scenarios such as unusually long or short eyes, as well as in steep or flat corneas.[4]

RELEVANCE OF REGRESSION FORMULAE IN CURRENT ERA

The SRK formula provides reasonable outcomes in average eyes within the normal range of AL, keratometry, and ACD/AL ratio. While the SRK II produces better outcomes in long and short eyes as compared to original SRK formula, the results are far from ideal.

SRK II formula still retains clinical significance in pediatric patients wherein biometry readings are often obtained on table during examination under anesthesia, using A-scan ultrasound for AL and hand-held keratometers for corneal power. Lee et al. compared visual outcomes of three formulae: SRK II, SRK-T, and Hoffer Q in pediatric patients undergoing IOL implantation for congenital cataract, and observed best predictive result with SRK II formula in patients <10 years of age.[14]

Regression formulae may also be preferred in diseased corneas, such as ectasia and corneal scarring. Thebpatiphat et al. compared SRK, SRK II, and SRK/T in patients with keratoconus undergoing cataract surgery with IOL implantation and observed the best predictive accuracy with SRK II in cases of mild keratoconus.[15]

CONCLUSION

Today, with the newer IOL power formulae and modern biometric techniques, the reported percentage of eyes within 0.5 D of target refraction is as high as 80–90%.[16] Though the SRK and SRK II formulae enjoyed immense popularity during the 1980s, they have been rendered rather obsolete in the current scenario owing to the advent of newer IOL power calculation formulae that produce much more accurate outcomes for all ranges of ALs.[17] Interestingly, several of the newer formulae combine modern regression models with other approaches such as theoretical mathematical model (SRK-T) or artificial intelligence (Hill-radial basis function calculator), validating its relevance in the current era.

REFERENCES

1. Retzlaff J. A new intraocular lens calculation formula. J Am Intraocul Implant Soc. 1980; 6:148-52.
2. Sanders DR, Kraff MC. Improvement of intraocular lens power calculation using empirical data. J Am Intraocul Implant Soc. 1980;6:263-7.
3. Ascaso FJ, Castillo JM, Cristóbal JA, Mínguez E, Palomar A. A comparative study of eight intraocular lens calculation formulas. Ophthalmologica. 1991;203:148-53.
4. Olsen T. Calculation of intraocular lens power: a review. Acta Ophthalmol Scand. 2007;85:472-85.
5. Menezo JL, Chaques V, Harto M. The SRK regression formula in calculating the dioptric power of intraocular lenses. Br J Ophthalmol. 1984;68:235-7.
6. Sanders DR, Retzlaff J, Kraff MC. Comparison of the SRK II formula and other second generation formulas. J Cataract Refract Surg. 1988;14:136-41.
7. Dang MS, Raj PP. SRK II formula in the calculation of intraocular lens power. Br J Ophthalmol. 1989;73:823-6.
8. Kora Y, Suzuki Y, Inatomi M, Ozawa T, Fukado Y. A simple modified SRK formula for severely myopic eyes. Ophthalmic Surg. 1990;21:266-71.
9. Kora Y, Totsuka N, Fukado Y, Marumori M, Yaguchi S. Modified SRK formula for axial myopia (24.5 mm < or = axial length < 27.0 mm). Ophthalmic Surg. 1992;23:603-7.
10. Retzlaff J. Posterior chamber implant power calculation: regression formulas. J Am Intraocul Implant Soc. 1980;6:268-70.
11. Olsen T, Thim K, Corydon L. Theoretical versus SRK I and SRK II calculation of intraocular lens power. J Cataract Refract Surg. 1990;16:217-25.
12. Olsen T, Thim K, Corydon L. Accuracy of the newer generation intraocular lens power calculation formulas in long and short eyes. J Cataract Refract Surg. 1991;17:187-93.
13. Sanders DR, Retzlaff JA, Kraff MC, Gimbel HV, Raanan MG. Comparison of the SRK/T formula and other theoretical and regression formulas. J Cataract Refract Surg. 1990;16:341-6.
14. Lee BJ, Lee S-M, Kim JH, Yu YS. Predictability of formulae for intraocular lens power calculation according to the age of implantation in paediatric cataract. Br J Ophthalmol. 2019;103:106-11.
15. Thebpatiphat N, Hammersmith KM, Rapuano CJ, Ayres BD, Cohen EJ. Cataract surgery in keratoconus. Eye Contact Lens. 2007;33:244-6.
16. Savini G, Hoffer KJ, Balducci N, Barboni P, Schiano-Lomoriello D. Comparison of formula accuracy for intraocular lens power calculation based on measurements by a swept-source optical coherence tomography optical biometer. J Cataract Refract Surg. 2020;46:27-33.
17. Gale RP, Saha N, Johnston RL. National biometry Audit II. Eye (London). 2006;20:25-8.

Vergence Formulae

INTRODUCTION

The first intraocular lens (IOL) power calculation formula introduced by Fyodorov in 1960s was based on the principle of theoretical refractive vergence. The formula incorporated axial length and keratometry for calculating the IOL power, while using a constant value for the pseudophakic anterior chamber depth (ACD) or the effective lens position (ELP), with the ACD value dependent on lens style and its placement in the eye. Subsequently, formulae such as Binkhorst II used variable ACD values based on axial length to improve outcomes.[1]

Modern-day vergence formulae incorporate multiple variables to accurately predict the ELP and provide enhanced refractive accuracy. They have evolved from traditional two-variable formulae including the Holladay 1, SRK-T, and Hoffer Q to elaborate seven-variable formulae such as the Holladay 2 formula, with excellent refractive predictability and wide usage amongst cataract surgeons over the decades.

We herein discuss the principle, different vergence formulae with the incorporated variables and their outcomes.

PRINCIPLE OF VERGENCE FORMULAE

Gaussian optics describes the behavior of light rays by using paraxial approximation, wherein only rays making a small angle with the optical axis are taken into consideration. The sine function in Snell's law is thus approximated by the argument, $\sin(\alpha) \approx \alpha$.

The vergence formula relies on Gaussian optics with the assumption that the image vergence is equal to the sum of the object and lens vergence. Vergence (V) at a given point may be calculated by the equation:

$$V = n/d$$

where n is the refractive index of the media and d is the distance of the object from the reference plane.[2]

The thin-lens formula is a simplified equation that assumes cornea and lens as single refracting plane without taking into account their thickness, curvature, or refractive index.[2] The refractive index of cornea is assumed to be 1.3375 with a fixed anterior-to-posterior curvature ratio. When a lens of power F is added to a bundle of rays of vergence V_1, the vergence V_2 of the rays leaving the lens can be calculated by equation:

$$V_2 = V_1 + F$$

Subtracting the vergence at the anterior part of IOL from the vergence at the posterior plane of the IOL gives the power of IOL needed for emmetropia inside the eye as described by the equation below:[2]

$$\text{IOL power} = n_2/(A - d) - 1/(1/K - d/n_1)$$

where A is axial length; K is corneal power, d is effective anterior chamber depth, n_1 is refractive index of anterior segment, and n_2 is refractive index of posterior segment.

The assumed position of the IOL or fictitious ELP in a thin-lens formula is represented by adjusted formula constants denoting the position of the lens of appropriate power that gives the eye the required target refraction. It can be reverse calculated from biometric parameters, power of IOL implanted and the postoperative refractive error, and does not necessarily coincide with the actual IOL position within the pseudophakic eye. Most vergence formulae used today including SRK/T, Hoffer Q, Holladay 1, and Haigis formulae are thin-lens formulae.

A thick-lens model considers the thickness, curvature, refractive index as well as the principal plane locations of cornea and lens. The ELP in a thick-lens model corresponds to the distance between the principal image plane of the cornea and the principal object plane of the IOL. The Emmetropia Verifying Optical (EVO) and Barrett Universal formulae are based on Gaussian thick-lens formula.[3]

■ VERGENCE FORMULAE

Modern-day vergence formulae may be classified based on the number of parameters or variables used to calculate the IOL power **(Table 1)**. Two-variable vergence formulae are often referred to as the third-generation formulae. Subsequent fourth-generation formulae include vergence formulae with additional variables and modifications of equation, such as Haigis, Holladay 2, and Barrett Universal II formulae. The ELP cannot be calculated directly and all vergence formulae use variables with a certain amount of regression to estimate the ELP.

Two-variable Vergence Formulae

The two-variable vergence formulae include the Holladay 1, SRK-T, and Hoffer Q.

TABLE 1: Salient features of various vergence formulae

IOL power calculation formula	Input variables	IOL constant	Clinical significance
Holladay 1	AL, K	Surgeon factor or SF	Best suited for eyes with AL range of 21.5–26.0 mm
SRK-T	AL, K	A-constant	Best suited for eyes with AL >26.0 mm
Hoffer Q	AL, K	pACD	Best suited for eyes with AL range of 20.0–22.0 mm
Haigis	AL, K, preoperative ACD	a0, a1, a2	Suited for axial lengths across the range with all three constants optimized
Barrett Universal II	AL, K, preoperative ACD, WTW, and LT	Lens Factor	Excellent results with axial lengths across all ranges
Holladay 2	AL, K, preoperative ACD, LT, corneal diameter, patient's age and preoperative refractive error	ACD	Good outcomes across all AL range; better outcomes in longer eyes

(ACD: anterior chamber depth; AL: axial length; IOL: intraocular lens; LT: lens thickness; K: keratometry; pACD: personalized anterior chamber depth; WTW: white to white)

The pseudophakic ACD or ELP is derived using axial length and keratometry. These formulae rely on the assumption that longer ALs and steeper K eyes are associated with deeper ELP. This assumption may not hold true for all eyes, especially in cases with extremes of axial lengths.

Holladay 1 Formula

Holladay 1 was the first two-variable vergence formula introduced in 1988. The ELP is calculated as the sum of anatomical ACD and the distance between the iris plane and the IOL's principal plane. The anatomical ACD is calculated as the sum of corneal height (distance from the corneal endothelium to the iris plane) and corneal thickness (0.56 mm). Corneal height is predicted using axial length and keratometry. The distance from the iris plane to the IOL's principal plane is termed *Surgeon Factor (SF)*, which is a personalized constant derived from a series of eyes operated by a single surgeon implanting a particular IOL model. The value for SF is obtained by postoperatively solving the formula in reverse using variables such as the preoperative corneal curvature, axial length, IOL power implanted, and the stabilized postoperative refraction. It aims to adjust for any consistent bias in the surgeon's results from any source.[4]

Clinical significance: The best results with Holladay 1 formula are seen in eyes with axial lengths ranging from 21.5 to 26.0 mm.[1,5]

SRK-T Formula

The *SRK/T formula* combines the original SRK regression method with a theoretical eye model. The formula used an *offset factor* analogous to the SF in Holladay 1 formula, referring to the distance between the iris plane and the IOL optical plane. The "offset factor" is derived from the $ACD_{constant}$, which is the ACD of a given IOL in an average eye for a surgeon. Postoperative ACD is calculated by adding this offset to the computed corneal height. Linear regression equation is derived which allows computation of $ACD_{constant}$ from the existing A constant. Additionally, the authors also use a different corneal refractive index and a correction factor for the retinal thickness.[6]

Clinical significance: The SRK-T formula shows best results in eyes with axial length >26.0 mm.[5,7] The performance of the formula is adversely affected by eyes that have flat or steep keratometry.[8]

Hoffer Q Formula

The *Hoffer Q formula* incorporates a *personalized ACD (pACD)*, axial length, and corneal curvature to calculate the ELP or pseudophakic ACD. The pACD is calculated by reverse calculating (like the SF) the ACD from the base Hoffer IOL power calculation formula for a given series of one IOL style. Factors for increasing the ACD corresponding to an increase in AL or keratometry are also included while computing the ELP. Additionally, a factor that moderated the change in ACD for extremely long (>26 mm) and short (<22 mm) eyes is incorporated into the formula. The ELP thus derived is included in the base Hoffer formula for calculating the IOL power.[1]

Clinical significance: Hoffer Q formula gives superior outcomes in shorter eyes with axial lengths ranging from 20.0 to 22.0 mm.[5] The accuracy of Hoffer Q formula is significantly affected by varying the AC depth.[8]

Three-variable Vergence Formulae

Three-variable vergence formulae include Haigis and Super Ladas formula.

Haigis Formula

Haigis formula utilizes the ACD and AL to predict the ELP. Thus AL, K, and ACD are required for IOL power calculation. Holladay 1, SRK-T, and Hoffer Q formulae use only one constant (e.g., SF, pACD, or A constant) to calculate the IOL power. In contrast, Haigis formula relies on three IOL and surgeon-specific constants, namely a0, a1, and a2. The constant a0 is derived from the classical A-constant provided by the IOL manufacturer while the constants a1 and a2 are based on the measured preoperative ACD and AL, respectively:

$$ELP = a_0 + a_1 \times ACD + a_2 \times AL$$

The three constants are a set of numbers which characterize each IOL type. For a given IOL, the value of these three constants is derived from the double regression analysis of ELP versus AL and ACD, where ELP is the measured pseudophakic ACD producing the true postoperative refraction.[9]

Clinical significance: Haigis formula with a0 optimized is suitable for eyes within the normal axial length range. For optimal performance of the formula including eyes at extremes of axial lengths, optimization of all three constants by the surgeon is recommended for a particular IOL type.

Super Ladas Formula

Ladas et al. devised a novel method of depicting the various formulae in three dimensions in 2015, and analysis of the 3-D representation helped discern areas where they were different or similar. Five formulae were graphed in three dimensions—Holladay 1, Holladay 1 with Wang-Koch modification (WKM), Hoffer Q, SRK-T, and Haigis. The most accurate portions of each formula were amalgamated to derive the Ladas super surface. The Ladas super-formula was derived from the Ladas supersurface with the aim of providing optimal IOL power for each individual eye. Inclusion of more formulae and optimization may help improve its accuracy further.[10]

Clinical significance: The formula can be applied to a wide range of eyes including the extremes of axial lengths.

Five-variable Vergence Formulae

Barrett Universal formula is a five-variable vergence formula with excellent refractive outcomes and predictability.

Barrett Universal Formula

Barrett Universal formula is based on a theoretical eye model and paraxial ray tracing in which the ACD is related to the AL and K. It uses five inputs for IOL power calculation-AL, K, ACD, white to white (WTW), and lens thickness (LT). It incorporates *"lens factor,"* which is associated with the physical position and location of principal planes of the IOL. ELP is derived from the ACD and the lens factor. The formula retains the concept of considering the ACD to consist of an anatomical axial-length-related component and a smaller IOL-related component inherent in the corneal height formula. The term "universal" in the formula emphasizes its suitability for all ranges of axial length.[11] In 2010, the Barrett Universal II (BU-II) formula, an updated version of Barrett Universal formula was introduced, which is freely available online at the official website of Asia Pacific Association of Cataract and Refractive Surgeons.[11,12]

Clinical significance: Barrett Universal II formula provides consistently accurate results in eyes with a wide range of axial lengths. It outperforms other formulae such as SRK/T, Haigis, Hoffer Q, Holladay 1, Holladay 2,

Olsen, and Hill RBF even in the extremely long eyes.[8,13,14] The formula has the advantage of being independently available, requiring minimal additional manipulation and no need for surgically induced astigmatism (SIA) data.[13]

Seven-variable Vergence Formula

Holladay 2 formula is a seven-variable vergence formula with more predictable outcomes as compared with Holladay 1.

Holladay 2 Formula

Holladay 2 formula is based on the theory that postoperative ACD can be more accurately estimated using biometric measurements of preoperative ACD, LT, corneal diameter, patient's age, and preoperative refractive error. These five parameters are incorporated in addition to AL and K in this seven-variable formula. It is available online on the Holladay IOL Consultant Program. The details of the formula have not been revealed by the author as yet.[15]

Clinical significance: The Holladay 2 formula has shown good outcomes in eyes with all ranges of axial lengths with more accurate outcomes in the longer AL group.[16] Studies have shown good accuracy with the formula even when parameters such as LT or preoperative refraction were not included.[16,17]

WANG–KOCH ADJUSTMENT IN IOL POWER CALCULATION

Wang-Koch adjustment method is used to optimize the AL while calculating IOL power in long eyes (AL >25 mm) to mitigate postoperative hyperopic surprise and achieve more accurate refractive outcomes. The authors evaluated five formulae—Holladay 1, Haigis, SRK/T, Hoffer Q, and Holladay 2. The optimized AL is derived from a regression equation for each of the formulae. The regression formula was developed by calculating the ideal AL which would produce zero manifest refraction, by back calculation using the manufacturer's lens constant and the postoperative manifest refraction obtained at 2.79 mm.[18] The authors have also suggested a modification to the original method, by using the ULIB IOL constants (instead of manufacturer's constants) and manifest refraction at 6 mm (instead of 2.79 mm).

OPTIMIZATION OF INTRAOCULAR LENS CONSTANTS

Optimization of IOL constants is the process by which a constant is refined for a particular surgical technique, lens, formula, surgeon, or measurement device based on previous outcomes. Systematic errors in IOL power calculation may arise due to different IOL types, biometry devices, and surgical techniques. Optimization may be performed with any formula, lens, or specific situation and is a method to eliminate the systematic prediction error of IOL power formulae and increase refractive predictability.[19] It is performed by an iterative method, wherein for specific IOL model and IOL calculation formula, the IOL constant for each eye is varied in 0.001 steps until the difference between the predicted and the actual spherical equivalent (SE) of the postoperative subjective refraction is zero. The optimized IOL constant is defined as the arithmetic mean of all individual IOL constants. It may be performed using optical biometers such as IOLMaster or online calculators. The use of optimized constants (such as SF, pACD, or A-constant) in IOL power formula rather than using the manufacturer's value is recommended to improve refractive outcomes while using these formulae for

IOL power calculation.[20] The minimum number of eyes required for IOL constant optimization varies from 50 to 250. Preferably, the eyes should have a postoperative visual acuity better than 6/12 and include a wide range of ALs while using the same biometry device. If a particular formula is intended for use in patients with a specific AL range, it is prudent to optimize the constant using eyes with AL in that range. The User group for Laser Interference Biometry (ULIB) constants were optimized based on a large number of preoperative and postoperative clinical data pooled from different surgical centers, albeit, without differentiating AL. For surgeons without a sufficient patient database to perform optimization, the ULIB constants are published and freely available on the website.[21]

DRAWBACKS OF VERGENCE FORMULAE

Intraocular lens power formulae based on Gaussian optics suffer certain drawbacks. The use of Gaussian optics is valid only if the rays of interest have a very small angle relative to the optical axis. The phenomenon of spherical aberration cannot be described by Gaussian optics. For example, the effective power of a spherical IOL will be stronger with larger pupil size due to positive spherical aberration. Gaussian optics-based formulae, however, fail to take this into account and are a poor approximation for the optics of human eye wherein the effective power of the IOL may vary with the change in pupil size.

Earlier IOL power calculation formula based on Gaussian optics assumed a constant postoperative ACD, which was inaccurate. Newer vergence formulae use ELP estimated from biometric parameters such as AL, K, and ACD, which may not correspond to the actual IOL position.[22]

CONCLUSION

Vergence formulae mark a significant advancement over the regression formulae with more accurate results, especially in extremes of axial length. Majority of conventional formulae give predictable outcomes in cases with axial length within the normal range of 22.0–24.5 mm. Vergence formulae have evolved from two-variable formulae tailored to the AL of the patient to formulae with multiple variables to predict the ELP, like Barrett II Universal and Holladay 2. Optimization of IOL constants helps further refine the refractive outcomes with these formulae.

REFERENCES

1. Hoffer KJ. The Hoffer Q formula: a comparison of theoretic and regression formulas. J Cataract Refract Surg. 1993;19:700-12.
2. Olsen T. Calculation of intraocular lens power: a review. Acta Ophthalmol Scand. 2007;85:472-85.
3. Gatinel D, Debellemanière G, Saad A, Dubois M, Rampat R. Determining the theoretical effective lens position of thick intraocular lenses for machine learning-based iol power calculation and simulation. Transl Vis Sci Technol. 2021;10:27.
4. Holladay JT, Prager TC, Chandler TY, Musgrove KH, Lewis JW, Ruiz RS. A three-part system for refining intraocular lens power calculations. J Cataract Refract Surg. 1988;14:17-24.
5. Aristodemou P, Knox Cartwright NE, Sparrow JM, Johnston RL. Formula choice: Hoffer Q, Holladay 1, or SRK/T and refractive outcomes in 8108 eyes after cataract surgery with biometry by partial coherence interferometry. J Cataract Refract Surg. 2011;37:63-71.
6. Retzlaff JA, Sanders DR, Kraff MC. Development of the SRK/T intraocular lens implant power calculation formula. J Cataract Refract Surg. 1990;16:333-40.

7. Narváez J, Zimmerman G, Stulting RD, Chang DH. Accuracy of intraocular lens power prediction using the Hoffer Q, Holladay 1, Holladay 2, and SRK/T formulas. J Cataract Refract Surg. 2006;32:2050-3.
8. Melles RB, Holladay JT, Chang WJ. Accuracy of intraocular lens calculation formulas. Ophthalmology. 2018;125:169-78.
9. Haigis W. Intraocular lens calculation after refractive surgery for myopia: Haigis-L formula. J Cataract Refract Surg. 2008;34: 1658-63.
10. Ladas JG, Siddiqui AA, Devgan U, Jun AS. A 3-D "super surface" combining modern intraocular lens formulas to generate a "super formula" and maximize accuracy. JAMA Ophthalmol. 2015;133:1431-6.
11. Barrett GD. An improved universal theoretical formula for intraocular lens power prediction. J Cataract Refract Surg. 1993;19: 713-20.
12. Biswas P, Batra S. Commentary: Barrett's Universal II formula: Time to change the old trends? Indian J Ophthalmol. 2020;68:64-5.
13. Roberts TV, Hodge C, Sutton G, Lawless M; contributors to the Vision Eye Institute IOL outcomes registry. Comparison of Hill-radial basis function, Barrett Universal and current third generation formulas for the calculation of intraocular lens power during cataract surgery. Clin Experiment Ophthalmol. 2018; 46:240-6.
14. Rong X, He W, Zhu Q, Qian D, Lu Y, Zhu X. Intraocular lens power calculation in eyes with extreme myopia: Comparison of Barrett Universal II, Haigis, and Olsen formulas. J Cataract Refract Surg 2019;45:732–737.
15. Hoffer KJ. Clinical results using the Holladay 2 intraocular lens power formula. J Cataract Refract Surg. 2000;26:1233-7.
16. Srivannaboon S, Chirapapaisan C, Chirapapaisan N, Lertsuwanroj B, Chongchareon M. Accuracy of Holladay 2 formula using IOLMaster parameters in the absence of lens thickness value. Graefes Arch Clin Exp Ophthalmol. 2013;251:2563-7.
17. Trivedi RH, Wilson ME, Reardon W. Accuracy of the Holladay 2 intraocular lens formula for pediatric eyes in the absence of preoperative refraction. J Cataract Refract Surg. 2011;37:1239-43.
18. Wang L, Shirayama M, Ma XJ, Kohnen T, Koch DD. Optimizing intraocular lens power calculations in eyes with axial lengths above 25.0 mm. J Cataract Refract Surg. 2011;37:2018-27.
19. Xia T, Martinez CE, Tsai LM. Update on Intraocular Lens Formulas and Calculations. Asia Pac J Ophthalmol (Phila). 2020;9: 186-93.
20. Aristodemou P, Knox Cartwright NE, Sparrow JM, Johnston RL. Intraocular lens formula constant optimization and partial coherence interferometry biometry: Refractive outcomes in 8108 eyes after cataract surgery. J Cataract Refract Surg. 2011;37:50-62.
21. Sheard R. Optimising biometry for best outcomes in cataract surgery. Eye (Lond) 2014;28:118-25.
22. Preussner P-R, Olsen T, Hoffmann P, Findl O. Intraocular lens calculation accuracy limits in normal eyes. J Cataract Refract Surg. 2008; 34:802-8.

CHAPTER 8

Aberrometry-based Formulae

■ INTRODUCTION

Optical methods for intraocular lens (IOL) power calculation are based on Gaussian optics or ray-tracing methods.[1] Conventional vergence formulae are based on Gaussian optics, from the older theoretical formulae given by Fyodorov and Binkhorst to the new-age Barrett universal II formula. They have inherent limitations in accurate prediction of effective lens position (ELP), and do not take into account the spherical aberrations of the eye. IOL power calculation has been revolutionized by the introduction of aberrometry-based formulae, which are not affected by the limitations of Gaussian optics-based formulae and are more predictable even in atypical scenarios. In this chapter, we evaluate the different ray-tracing-based IOL power formulae and intraoperative aberrometry for IOL power calculation, including their basic principles, advantages, and clinical significance.

■ PRINCIPLE OF RAY-TRACING FORMULAE

The ray-tracing method calculates the path of a single ray of light through an optical system, by applying the Snell's law to each refracting surface that the ray passes through. The complex calculations are performed using computers, and IOL power is calculated based on true geometric data including distances, local radii of all refracting surfaces, and the corresponding refractive indices.[2]

The ray-tracing method does not rely on paraxial approximations unlike the vergence formulae and takes into account the asphericity and aberrations of lens and cornea. The postoperative IOL position denotes the geometrical position of IOL, which is estimated using preoperative anterior chamber depth (ACD), lens thickness (LT), and lens position as well as the IOL characteristics, rather than the fictitious ELP in thin-lens formulae.[2,3] **Table 1** compares the basic principle and salient features of Gaussian optics-based thin-lens formulae and ray-tracing-based formulae.

■ RAY-TRACING FORMULAE

The Olsen formula and the IOL power calculation software, namely Okulix and PhacoOptics, are based on numerical ray tracing. More recently a ray-tracing-based formula, termed the "O formula," using swept-source anterior segment optical coherence tomography (ASOCT)-based biometer, was proposed by Goto et al.[4]

Olsen Formula

Olsen formula was originally described as a paraxial thick-lens formula.[5] Subsequently, exact ray tracing was used to correct the assumptions of the paraxial model, thus

TABLE 1: Comparison of salient features of Gaussian optics thin-lens formulae and ray-tracing formulae

Paraxial formulae based on thin-lens model	Ray-tracing formulae
Consider the paraxial optical path only	Use Snell's law to calculate path of a single ray of light through an optical system
Do not account for the change in corneal curvature with pupil diameter owing to its aberration profile	Take into account pupil diameter, corneal irregularity, and corneal aberration profile
Cornea and lens are assumed to be single refracting surfaces without any thickness	Approach the lens and cornea as thick lens having two surfaces and a finite thickness and refractive index
Assume fixed ratio between anterior and posterior corneal curvature	Take the curvature of the anterior and posterior corneal surfaces and corneal thickness into account
IOL position is denoted by a fictitious ELP represented by a constant rather than an actual physical dimension	Postoperative IOL position is an actual physical dimension which is predicted on the basis of preoperative parameters, such as ACD and LT
Most formulae use keratometry values from the central 2–3 mm of cornea	Linkage of ray-tracing software to topographers or tomographers allows the use of corneal surface information from a wider area

(ACD: anterior chamber depth; ELP: effective lens position; IOL: intraocular lens; LT: lens thickness)

combining both models to estimate the true physical dimensions of the eye's optical system while avoiding the errors of a thin-lens formula.[6]

Olsen formula comes in two versions: The four-factor version also known as the Olsen$_{standalone}$ (accessed via PhacoOptics software), which uses axial length (AL), keratometry (K), LT, and ACD for ELP estimation, and the two-factor version based on the C-constant, which uses preoperative ACD and LT only for ELP estimation and is installed on optical biometers, such as Lenstar LS 900. The C-constant defines the final IOL position from the preoperative ACD and LT. The postoperative IOL position is given by the equation:

$$IOL_c = ACD_{pre} + C \times LT_{pre}$$

where IOL_c = center of the IOL, ACD_{pre} = preoperative anterior chamber depth, LT_{pre} = preoperative crystalline lens thickness, and C = constant related to the IOL type that reflects the average contraction of the capsular bag around the IOL in the axial direction.

The value of the constant C was derived by evaluating the ACD before and after cataract surgery in 2,043 patients:[7]

$$C = (Postoperative\ ACD + 1/2 \times TIOL - Preoperative\ ACD)/Preoperative\ LT$$

where, LT = lens thickness, TIOL = thickness of the IOL, and ACD = anterior chamber depth.

The value of "C" varies with different types of IOLs based on their design and material. The Olsen formula bases its ELP predictions on the actual measurements of the postoperative IOL position unlike in Gaussian optics formulae where it is a back-calculated variable, thus segregating the estimation of the physical IOL position from the optics of the IOL power calculation formula.[7]

Studies have suggested the four-factor version to be more accurate than two-factor version.[8,9] The other inputs for the formula include age and central corneal thickness (optional).[8] The use of Olsen formula also requires six lens constants to be filled-in by the user. Five of these constants are related to IOL manufacturing specifications, namely LT, index of refraction, anterior radius, posterior radius, and spherical aberration while the sixth is for ACD.[8]

Numerical Ray-tracing Software for Intraocular Lens Power Calculation

Okulix (Panopsis GmbH, Mainz, Germany) and PhacoOptics (IOL Innovations ApS, Aarhus, Denmark) are the two commercially available ray-tracing softwares for IOL power calculation. Both softwares can be linked to various topographers, tomographers, and optical biometers as listed further. **Table 2** summarizes the characteristics of Okulix ray-tracing software and Olsen formula.

The Okulix software was developed by Dr Paul-Rolf Preussner for IOL power calculation by the means of ray tracing using a pseudophakic eye model. It can be linked to biometers such as Haag-Streit Lenstar, Oculus Pentacam, Tracey iTrace, Zeimer Galilei G6, Tomey CASIA ASOCT, or Heidelberg Anterion. Inputs include AL, corneal topography and pachymetry, preoperative ACD, and LT (when available), as well as the IOL-related information contained within the software database such as the anterior and posterior curvature radii, asphericity, central thickness, and refractive index. These inputs are used to calculate the IOL power that gives the best focus or the smallest simulated image of a Landolt C on the fovea. The AL is entered manually or directly transferred in from a connected device. As the device uses optical length rather than ultrasonic length, it transforms the values incorporated from the measuring device. The software also considers diffraction of rays at the pupillary aperture and the effect of oblique incidence of light rays or the Stiles–Crawford effect. The calculated position of the IOL denotes its geometrical position, i.e., the distance between the posterior corneal apex and the anterior IOL apex. Model calculation (based on linear regression) is used to estimate the

TABLE 2: Ray-tracing-based IOL power calculation formulae

Formula	Principle	Input variables	Outcomes
Olsen formula (Incorporated in PhacoOptics software)	Combines exact ray tracing with paraxial thick-lens model	Age, CCT (optional), 6 constants along with AL, K, ACD, LT in 4-factor version (ACD, LT in 2-factor version)	• Excellent outcomes in normal eyes—up to 81% of eyes with refractive predictive error within 0.5 D. Comparable to Barrett Universal II, Kane formula • Olsen four-factor formula second most accurate (to Kane formula) in normal as well as short and long AL subgroups
Okulix ray-tracing software	Numerical ray tracing using a pseudophakic eye model	AL, K/corneal topography, CCT, ACD, and LT (when available), and IOL-related information (stored in software)	• Excellent outcomes in normal eyes, up to 82% of eyes with refractive predictive error within 0.5 D. Comparable to Barrett Universal II, Kane formula • Excellent outcomes in post-LVC eyes—up to 85% eyes with refractive predictive error <0.5 D

(ACD: anterior chamber depth; CCT: central corneal thickness; IOL: intraocular lens; K: keratometry; LT: lens thickness; LVC: laser vision correction)

most probable IOL position, and the actual IOL position may be influenced by additional variables, such as individual capsular shrinkage.[10]

The PhacoOptics software developed by Dr T Olsen incorporates the four-factor Olsen formula in its standalone version. It can be linked to Lenstar (Haag-Streit), Oculus Pentacam, Zeiss IOL-Master 700, Topcon Aladdin, Tomey OA-2000, and Zeimer Galilie G6. Ray-tracing software linked to ASOCT-based tomographers are advantageous in corneal opacities as ASOCT may better measure the anterior and posterior curvature as compared to Scheimpflug-based devices.[11]

■ OUTCOMES

Ray-tracing-based formulae have shown excellent outcomes in normal eyes comparable to other modern formulae, such as Kane or Barrett Universal II, with 72–81% of eyes having a predictive error within 0.5 D.[9,11-13] It is advantageous over the conventional formulae in atypical scenarios, such as the extremes of ALs, post-laser vision correction (LVC), or irregular corneas.

Post-laser Vision Correction

Ray-tracing method is not affected by the keratometric index error in postrefractive surgery eyes. The IOL position is calculated based on the preoperative ACD and LT and does not rely on keratometry. Moreover, when used with topographers, the corneal curvature is measured over the entire 3–7 mm zone and is not limited to 3 mm zone unlike the simulated K values.[14] In post-LVC patients, ray-tracing-based IOL calculation with anterior corneal surface topographer alone resulted in 42–84% of eyes with a prediction error within 0.5 D.[15-17] With the use of tomographers such as Anterion ASOCT, which measure both anterior and posterior corneal curvature, about 88% of the eyes were within 0.5 D of target.[10] A recent network meta-analysis observed up to 85% of eyes within 0.5 D of prediction using ray-tracing-based formulae in post-LVC eyes.[18,19]

Extremes of Axial Lengths

Ray-tracing formulae estimate the actual physical IOL position taking into account the variation in anterior segment anatomy rather than estimating a fictitious ELP, which results in excellent outcomes in extremes of AL.[7]

Olsen formula outperforms advanced modern formulae, such as Kane, EVO, and Barrett Universal II formula in long eyes, with a prediction error of <0.5 D in 70–85% of eyes.[8,9,20] For short eyes, Olsen formula outperforms two-variable vergence formulae but not the modern formulae, such as Kane and Barrett Universal II formula.[21] Studies report 53–71% of eyes with a refractive prediction error within 0.5 D.[8,21,22] Olsen formulae and Okulix software have emerged as one of the most accurate formulae in eyes with extremes of AL.[9,23]

Toric/Aspheric Intraocular Lenses

Ray-tracing approach allows the prediction of postoperative refractive aberrations and retinal image quality produced by the interaction between IOL power, asphericity, toricity, and natural corneal aberrations, thus aiding the surgeon in choosing the most suitable IOL type and power.[24]

■ INTRAOPERATIVE ABERROMETRY

Intraoperative aberrometry provides intraoperative refraction in real time, which in conjunction with preoperative biometry is used to refine the calculated IOL power and axis. It was first made commercially available on ORange wavefront aberrometer (WaveTec Vision Inc., Aliso Viejo, California, USA). Subsequently Optiwave Refractive Analysis (ORA) System (Alcon Laboratories, Inc., Fort Worth, Texas, USA) was introduced.

Principle

The ORA system utilizes a form of wavefront analysis called Talbot–Moiré interferometry, which combines a Talbot diffraction effect with a Moiré pattern.[25] Optical wavefront from the device passes through a pair of gratings set a particular distance and angle apart. Diffraction produces a fringe pattern, which is projected on to the eye and causes distortions. The aberrometer analysis of these distortions or aberrations is used to perform refractive calculations using a proprietary analysis system.[26] Based on the refractive analysis, the aberrometer suggests the appropriate power and toricity of an IOL to be implanted in an aphakic IOL or whether an implanted toric IOL should be rotated from its current alignment. The aberrometer is linked to AnalyzOR, a cloud-based database of preoperative, intraoperative, and postoperative refractive data.

Limitations

The accuracy of intraoperative aberrometry measurements tends to be affected by several factors. These include the pressure on the globe determined by the positioning of the lid speculum, presence of viscoelastic in the anterior chamber, ocular surface irregularity, intraocular pressure, corneal wound integrity, wound hydration, and vitreous hydration. Proper fixation by the patient is a prerequisite for reliable measurements, which makes it unfeasible in uncooperative patients or those having involuntary eye movements. Moreover, surgical time is prolonged, which may have implications on operating room efficiency as well as surgical cost.[26]

Clinical Application and Outcomes

Intraoperative aberrometry is a useful adjunct to refine IOL power calculation and on-table alignment. In normal eyes, comparable outcomes are observed with intraoperative aberrometry, Barrett Universal II and Hill-RBF 2.0, with 82, 84, and 83% of eyes within 0.5 D of refractive target, respectively.[27] Advantage is observed in the cases with discrepancy in intraoperative aberrometry and preoperatively calculated IOL power, especially if IOL power calculated using ORA is higher.[28]

Intraoperative aberrometry measures both the total corneal as well as surgically induced astigmatism, and results in lower postoperative residual astigmatism in patients undergoing toric IOL implantation.[29] In the extremes of AL, the results are comparable to modern IOL power formula, such as Hill-RBF 2.0 and Barrett Universal II.[27] In eyes with a history of myopic laser ablative surgery, intraoperative aberrometry is more accurate than Haigis L or Shammas PL; however, the outcomes are comparable to Barrett True-K formula with 54–68% eyes within 0.5 D of target.[30,31] Intraoperative aberrometry was found to be comparable to Barrett True-K formula in post-hyperopic corneal ablative surgery.[32] Similarly, in post-radial keratotomy (RK) patients, intraoperative aberrometry failed to demonstrate a significant advantage over the Barrett True-K formula with 36–55.3% eyes having target refractive error within 0.5 D.[32]

■ CONCLUSION

Ray-tracing-based formulae have emerged as a promising alternative to mitigate the limitations of Gaussian optics formulae, with excellent outcomes in normal eyes and extremes of AL.[9] More recently, incorporation of machine-learning algorithms for predicting postoperative ACD in Okulix software has further increased the prediction accuracy, particularly in patients with extremes of ALs.[33] Despite the promising results, ray-tracing-based formulae software such as PhacoOptics and Okulix have not attained widespread usage owing to the cost of acquiring the formulae for clinical use. Intraoperative aberrometry is a useful adjunct for validating or modifying the IOL power but has not supplanted a thorough preoperative patient workup and planning.

■ REFERENCES

1. Olsen T. Calculation of intraocular lens power: a review. Acta Ophthalmol Scand. 2007;85(5):472-85.
2. Preussner PR, Wahl J, Lahdo H, Dick B, Findl O. Ray tracing for intraocular lens calculation. J Cataract Refract Surg. 2002;28(8):1412-9.
3. Preussner PR, Olsen T, Hoffmann P, Findl O. Intraocular lens calculation accuracy limits in normal eyes. J Cataract Refract Surg. 2008;34(5):802-8.
4. Goto S, Maeda N, Ohnuma K, Lawu T, Kawasaki R, Koh S, et al. Preliminary demonstration of a novel intraocular lens power calculation: the O formula. J Cataract Refract Surg. 2022;48(11):1305-11.
5. Olsen T. Theoretical approach to intraocular lens calculation using Gaussian optics. J Cataract Refract Surg. 1987;13(2):141-5.
6. Olsen T, Funding M. Ray-tracing analysis of intraocular lens power in situ. J Cataract Refract Surg. 2012;38(4):641-7.
7. Olsen T, Hoffmann P. C constant: new concept for ray tracing-assisted intraocular lens power calculation. J Cataract Refract Surg. 2014;40(5):764-73.
8. Cooke DL, Cooke TL. Prediction accuracy of preinstalled formulas on 2 optical biometers. J Cataract Refract Surg. 2016;42(3):358-62.
9. Melles RB, Kane JX, Olsen T, Chang WJ. Update on intraocular lens calculation formulas. Ophthalmology. 2019;126(9):1334-5.
10. Gjerdrum B, Gundersen KG, Lundmark PO, Aakre BM. Refractive precision of ray tracing IOL calculations based on OCT data versus traditional IOL calculation formulas based on reflectometry in patients with a history of laser vision correction for myopia. Clin Ophthalmol. 2021;15:845-57.
11. Minami K, Kataoka Y, Matsunaga J, Ohtani S, Honbou M, Miyata K. Ray-tracing intraocular lens power calculation using anterior segment optical coherence tomography measurements. J Cataract Refract Surg. 2012;38(10):1758-63.
12. Hoffmann PC, Lindemann CR. Intraocular lens calculation for aspheric intraocular lenses. J Cataract Refract Surg. 2013;39(6):867-72.
13. Connell BJ, Kane JX. Comparison of the Kane formula with existing formulas for intraocular lens power selection. BMJ Open Ophthalmol. 2019;4(1):e000251.
14. Lazaridis A, Schraml F, Preußner PR, Sekundo W. Predictability of intraocular lens power calculation after small-incision lenticule extraction for myopia. J Cataract Refract Surg. 2021;47(3):304-10.
15. Saiki M, Negishi K, Kato N, Torii H, Dogru M, Tsubota K. Ray tracing software for intraocular lens power calculation after corneal excimer laser surgery. Jpn J Ophthalmol. 2014;58(3):276-81.
16. Canovas C, van der Mooren M, Rosén R, Piers PA, Wang L, Koch DD, et al. Effect of the equivalent refractive index on intraocular lens power prediction with ray tracing after myopic laser in situ keratomileusis. J Cataract Refract Surg. 2015;41(5):1030-7.
17. Savini G, Bedei A, Barboni P, Ducoli P, Hoffer KJ. Intraocular lens power calculation by ray-tracing after myopic excimer laser surgery. Am J Ophthalmol. 2014;157(1):150-3.
18. Gale RP, Saldana M, Johnston RL, Zuberbuhler B, McKibbin M. Benchmark standards for refractive outcomes after NHS cataract surgery. Eye (London). 2009;23(1):149-52.

19. Wen D, Yu J, Zeng Z, McAlinden C, Hu L, Feng K, et al. Network meta-analysis of no-history methods to calculate intraocular lens power in eyes with previous myopic laser refractive surgery. J Refract Surg. 2020; 36(7):481-90.
20. Ma Y, Xiong R, Liu Z, Young CA, Wu Y, Zheng D, et al. Network meta-analysis of IOL power calculation formula accuracy in 1,016 eyes with long axial length. Am J Ophthalmol. 2024;257:178-86.
21. Kane JX, Chang DF. Intraocular lens power formulas, biometry, and intraoperative aberrometry: A review. Ophthalmology. 2021;128(11):e94-114.
22. Kane JX, Melles RB. Intraocular lens formula comparison in axial hyperopia with a high-power intraocular lens of 30 or more diopters. J Cataract Refract Surg. 2020;46(9):1236-9.
23. Luo Y, Li H, Gao L, Du J, Chen W, Gao Y, et al. Comparing the accuracy of new intraocular lens power calculation formulae in short eyes after cataract surgery: a systematic review and meta-analysis. Int Ophthalmol. 2022;42(6):1939-56.
24. Pérez-Merino P, Aramberri J, Quintero AV, Rozema JJ. Ray tracing optimization: a new method for intraocular lens power calculation in regular and irregular corneas. Sci Rep. 2023;13(1):4555.
25. Sarver EJ, Van Heugten TY, Padrick TD, Hall MT. Astigmatic refraction using peaks of the interferogram Fourier transform for a Talbot Moiré interferometer. J Refract Surg. 2007;23(9):972-7.
26. Hemmati HD, Gologorsky D, Pineda R. Intraoperative wavefront aberrometry in cataract surgery. Semin Ophthalmol. 2012; 27(5-6):100-6.
27. Raufi N, James C, Kuo A, Vann R. Intraoperative aberrometry vs modern preoperative formulas in predicting intraocular lens power. J Cataract Refract Surg. 2020; 46(6):857-61.
28. Cionni RJ, Dimalanta R, Breen M, Hamilton C. A large retrospective database analysis comparing outcomes of intraoperative aberrometry with conventional preoperative planning. J Cataract Refract Surg. 2018; 44(10): 1230-5.
29. Yesilirmak N, Palioura S, Culbertson W, Yoo SH, Donaldson K. Intraoperative wavefront aberrometry for toric intraocular lens placement in eyes with a history of refractive surgery. J Refract Surg. 2016;32(1):69-70.
30. Ianchulev T, Hoffer KJ, Yoo SH, Chang DF, Breen M, Padrick T, et al. Intraoperative refractive biometry for predicting intraocular lens power calculation after prior myopic refractive surgery. Ophthalmology. 2014; 121(1):56-60.
31. Kauffmann T, Bodanowitz S, Hesse L, Kroll P. Corneal reinnervation after photorefractive keratectomy and laser in situ keratomileusis: an in vivo study with a confocal videomicroscope. Ger J Ophthalmol. 1996;5(6): 508-12.
32. Gouvea L, Sioufi K, Brown CE, Waring Iv G, Chamon W, Rocha KM. Refractive accuracy of barrett true-K vs intraoperative aberrometry for IOL power calculation in post-corneal refractive surgery eyes. Clin Ophthalmol. 2021;15:4305-15.
33. Li T, Reddy A, Stein JD, Nallasamy N. Ray tracing intraocular lens calculation performance improved by AI-powered postoperative lens position prediction. Br J Ophthalmol. 2023;107(4):483-7.

CHAPTER 9

Artificial Intelligence in Intraocular Lens Power Calculation

■ INTRODUCTION

Artificial intelligence (AI) is increasingly finding a role in health care, with an application in fields with image-based diagnostics. In ophthalmology, AI has been utilized for automated analysis of fundus images, optical coherence tomography images, and visual fields, and various clinical trials have established its efficacy in the diagnosis of diabetic retinopathy. The utilization of AI in cataract surgery is being explored in preoperative diagnosis, intraocular lens (IOL) power calculation, and predicting postoperative refraction.

Refractive outcomes after cataract surgery have improved greatly with new-generation IOL power calculation formulae, with nearly 50–70% eyes within 0.5 D and 80–90% eyes within 1.0 D of the target refraction.[1-3] New-generation formulae incorporate multiple variables to effectively predict the IOL power and effective lens position (ELP); however, they cannot account for individual variations and may not be as accurate in all patients.

Artificial intelligence is being used in IOL power calculation to customize the IOL power, taking into account a host of variables to enhance the refractive predictability and accuracy. A number of formulae incorporating AI are now available for clinical use, including the Hill-radial basis function (RBF) 3.0, Ladas Super Formula 2.0, Kane formula, etc., and their outcomes are superior or comparable to the latest-generation conventional IOL power calculation formulae. We herein evaluate the applications of AI in IOL power calculation and critically evaluate its utility in enhancing refractive outcomes.

■ ARTIFICIAL INTELLIGENCE METHODOLOGY AND TECHNIQUES

The AI approaches utilized in ophthalmology are based on machine learning or deep learning. Machine learning involves complex algorithms to analyze large, labeled datasets and identify patterns in the data to enhance diagnostics. Statistical methods are utilized to learn from the outcomes, and the accuracy of AI increases with larger datasets. Deep learning is an advanced form of machine learning, with complex multilayered programming akin to the human brain, which can analyze both labeled and unlabeled data.

The machine-learning models that have been utilized for IOL power calculation include artificial neural networks (ANNs), eXtreme Gradient Boosting (XGBoost), and support vector regression (SVR) **(Table 1)**.[4] They are nonlinear, regression supervised learning methods which utilize the outcome data to predict or adjust outcomes. ANN is composed of nodes and layers akin to the human brain, and each layer is built up by

TABLE 1: Artificial intelligence machine-learning algorithms used in IOL power calculation

Algorithm	Description
ANN	• Consists of nodes and layers—each node is a nonlinear filter; layer built up by parallel nodes • Input goes through a network of nodes and the weights of the connections learned by training the ANN model • Combination of nodes reveals the nonlinear relationship between the inputs and output to predict the outcome
SVR	• Creates a predictive model based on both input variables and outcome data • Predicts the nonlinear relationship between the input variables and outcome as a continuous variable rather than a binary classification
XGBoost	• Gradient boosting method • Assembles many weak prediction models used in decision trees • Combines many decision trees to reveal the relationship between the input variables and output

(ANN: artificial neural network; SVR: support vector regression; XGBoost: extreme gradient boosting)

parallel nodes. The nonlinear relationship between the input variables and output is revealed by the combination of these nodes and used to predict the outcome. XGBoost combines multiple decision trees to analyze the relation between the input variables and the output. SVR incorporates both the input variables and outcome data to create a predictive model.

ARTIFICIAL INTELLIGENCE-BASED INTRAOCULAR LENS POWER CALCULATION FORMULAE

Various AI-based IOL power calculation formulae are available for clinical use and include the Hill-RBF 3.0, Kane, Ladas, Pearl-DGS, Hoffer Q Savini/Taroni (Hoffer QST) formulae **(Table 2)**. These formulae have superior refractive outcomes compared with conventional IOL power calculation formulae, with approximately 90% of eyes achieving postoperative refraction within 0.5 D of the intended target. In addition, various studies have evaluated the application of machine-learning algorithms on existing IOL power calculation methods and observed enhanced accuracy and refractive predictability.[5-7]

Hill-Radial Basis Function 3.0

The Hill-RBF was the first AI-based formula available for commercial use. It is a purely AI-based formula created using a RBF network (type of neural network), and the input variables include axial length, keratometry, and anterior chamber depth.[8] The Hill-RBF calculator has been developed by Dr Warren Hill in association with Haag-Streit Switzerland and Mathworks, and is freely available for online use.

The original Hill-RBF formula was based on the dataset of 3,400 surgical cases performed by high-volume surgeons around the world. The Hill-RBF 2.0 used an expanded dataset of 12,000 eyes collected from the Lenstar biometer (Haag-Streit) and implanted with an SN60WL IOL (Alcon).

The Hill-RBF 3.0 is the most recent version of the calculator with a further expanded dataset. Hill-RBF 3.0 provides calculations for biconvex IOLs from +34.00 D to +6.00 D and for meniscus design IOLs from +5.00 D to –5.00 D. It is based on eight variables, including lens thickness, white-to-white (WTW), central corneal thickness, and gender.

The formula uses AI for pattern recognition and data interpolation to predict the IOL power and postoperative refraction directly based on the fixed dataset, without the need

CHAPTER 9: Artificial Intelligence in Intraocular Lens Power Calculation

TABLE 2: Artificial intelligence-based IOL power calculation formulae

Formula	Principle	Input variables	Availability	Outcomes
Hill-RBF (Version 3.0-2020, Version 2.0-2018, Version 1.0-2016)	AI RBF network	• AL, K, ACD, A-constant, LT, WTW, CCT, and gender • Postoperative refractive target	• Incorporated in Lenstar and the Eyestar biometers • Free online calculator	• Prediction error within 0.5 D in over 90% of eyes with Hill-RBF 3.0 • More accurate than previous versions of Hill-RBF formula • Superior/comparable to modern IOL power calculation formulae in various studies
Kane formula	Hybrid AI formula—combines regression and AI techniques	• AL, K, ACD, LT, CCT, gender, and A-constant • Postoperative refractive target	• Preinstalled on Veracity Surgery Planner (Zeiss) wand EQ Workplace (Zeiss) • Free online calculator	Superior/comparable to Barrett Universal II in various studies. Excellent outcomes in long (>26 mm) and short eyes
Ladas Super Formula 2.0	• AI • Applied on original Ladas Super Formula	• Formulae incorporated in Ladas Super Formula include SRK/T, Hoffer Q, Holladay 1, Holladay with WK adjustment, and Haigis • Postoperative refractive target	Online calculator allows application of their AI algorithm (PLUS algorithm) to any static formula	• Limited literature • Promising outcomes in published studies
Hoffer QST	AI	AL, K, ACD, pACD, and postoperative refractive target	Installed on Optopol biometer	• Limited literature • Promising outcomes in published studies
PEARL-DGS	Hybrid AI-based thick-lens formula	AL, K, ACD, LT, WTW, CCT, A constant, and postoperative refractive target	Uses python code-easily available	• Limited literature • Promising outcomes in published studies
Zeiss AI IOL calculator	AI and paraxial ray tracing	• Integrated into Zeiss VERACITY surgical planner • Utilizes 16,000 IOL parameters to refine the predicted IOL power for each IOL model	Exclusively available on ZEISS VERACITY Surgery Planner	• Limited literature • Promising outcomes in published studies

(ACD: anterior chamber depth; AI: artificial intelligence; AL: axial length; CCT: central corneal thickness; Hoffer QST: Hoffer Q Savini/Taroni; K: keratometry; LT: lens thickness; PEARL-DGS: prediction enhanced by artificial intelligence and output linearization-Debellemanière, Gatinel, and Saad; PLUS: Precision Ladas Universal Super; RBF: radial basis function; SRK/T: Sanders–Retzlaff–Kraff theoretic; WK: Wang Koch; WTW: white-to-white) for prediction of ELP or vergence. It also incorporates a "boundary model" that detects outliers (out of bounds) when the predicted power is likely to be unreliable.

It has led to an increase in postoperative refractive accuracy, with nearly 90% eyes within 0.5 D of predicted refraction. The limitation of the formula is that it is based on a fixed dataset, and the results may not be applicable in different populations. Unreliable results are obtained where there is paucity of data. Additional variables cannot be incorporated in the present calculator; a new dataset would be required for the same.

Kane Formula

The Kane formula is also based on "big data" and was created using large data sets of approximately 30,000 eyes from high-volume surgeons. It is a combination formula based on theoretical optics and a thin-lens formula.[9] Both regression analysis and AI techniques are utilized to predict the IOL power. The variations induced by IOL design and power range are taken into account by the Kane formula.

The parameters used in Kane formula include axial length, keratometry, anterior chamber depth, lens thickness, central corneal thickness, and biological sex.

Ladas Super Formula 2.0

The Ladas Super Formula is an amalgamation of five conventional IOL power calculation formulae—Hoffer Q, Holladay 1, Holladay 1 with Koch adjustment, Haigis, and Sanders-Retzlaff-Kraff theoretic (SRK/T). Nonlinear regression modeling and 3D surface plotting techniques are employed to improve the refractive predictions. The super formula incorporates the ideal segments from each of the existing formulae and uses the ideal IOL formula for an individual eye.[10]

Ladas Super Formula 2.0 uses the original super formula as the framework. It incorporates AI algorithms and big-data approach to predict the displacement between the existing formula and perfect outcomes and make adjustments to the tune of 0.2 D in the recommended IOL power. Multiple variables can be taken into account using this approach to enhance the accuracy of refractive outcomes; in addition, unlike Hill-RBF formula, there is no risk of "out of bounds" result as it is based on the framework of an existing formula.

Precision Ladas Universal Super (PLUS) algorithm allows the application of the advanced AI algorithm developed by Ladas to any existing formula in order to increase its accuracy.[4]

ZEISS Artificial Intelligence Intraocular Lens Calculator

The ZEISS AI IOL Calculator incorporates a large dataset of over 100,000 eyes, collected mostly from ZEISS VERACITY Surgery Planner users. The calculator utilizes AI algorithms and paraxial ray tracing to improve surgical outcomes. More than 16,000 IOL parameters are incorporated to refine the predicted IOL power for each IOL model and also predict the postoperative IOL position. The continual expansion of the dataset allows constant refinement of the calculator with improved performance and accuracy.[11]

PEARL-DGS

PEARL is an acronym for Prediction Enhanced by ARtificial intelligence and output Linearization and DGS refers to the formula developers—Debellemanière, Gatinel, and Saad. PEARL-DGS is an open-source hybrid AI-based thick-lens formula that uses two algorithms to enhance predictive accuracy.[12] Machine-learning modeling and output linearization are utilized to effectively predict the posterior corneal radius and the theoretical internal lens position, as well as perform adjustments for extremes of biometry. The input variables include axial length, keratometry, anterior chamber depth, lens thickness, WTW, and central corneal thickness.

Hoffer Q/Savini/Taroni

The Hoffer Q/Savini/Taroni (Hoffer QST) formula employs AI algorithms on the existing Hoffer Q formula to predict the ELP and improve refractive accuracy in long eyes.[13]

CLINICAL OUTCOMES

The AI-based IOL power calculation formulae are equivalent or slightly superior to the newer generation IOL power calculation formulae such as Olsen, Holladay 2, and Barrett Universal II.[1,14,15] In addition, improved refractive results are observed when AI algorithms are applied to the conventional IOL power calculation formulae.[4,16]

Darcy et al. evaluated the accuracy of nine IOL power calculation formulae based on the outcomes of 10,930 eyes and observed the lowest mean absolute prediction error with the Kane formula. The percentage of eyes within 0.5 D of the target refraction was 72% with Kane formula, 71.2% with Hill-RBF 2.0, 70.6% with Olsen, 71% with Holladay 2, 70.7% with Barrett II, 69.1% with SRK/T, 69% with Haigis, and 68.1% with Hoffer Q.[14]

A review of eight modern IOL power calculation formulae observed superior refractive outcomes with Kane and Barrett Universal-II formulae over the entire axial length spectrum, with Kane formula being most accurate in longer axial lengths of >26 mm.[17]

Nemeth et al. observed the highest accuracy of prediction error with the Hill-RBF 2.0 formula, with Kane, PEARL-DGS, and Barrett Universal II formulae having similar accuracy.[15] In contrast, Kane et al. observed Barrett Universal II formula to be the most accurate with significantly less mean absolute error as compared with Hill-RBF and Ladas Super Formula.[1]

FALLACIES OF ARTIFICIAL INTELLIGENCE

Majority of the commonly used AI-based IOL power calculation formulae are devised using machine-learning models on large datasets, with the outcomes used for analysis obtained from Caucasian eyes. These formulae may not be as accurate when applied to populations with different ethnicities and race. Geometric or anatomical differences in different patient groups will lead to variations in the ocular optics and may adversely impact the predictability of AI-based formulae.

Another limitation of AI-based formulae is unreliable or out-of-bounds results in certain types of eyes due to a sparsity of data, such as in eyes with extremes of axial length. Present-day AI-based formulae may result in refractive surprises in highly myopic eyes.[1,18] In addition, the formulae may in itself have input limits of certain variables such as axial length and target refraction. For instance, both Kane and Hill-RBF 3.0 have an axial length limit of 35 mm. Hill-RBF 3.0 has target refraction limit ranging from –2.5 D to +1.0 D.

WHAT THE FUTURE HOLDS

The AI-based IOL power calculation formulae display a trend toward enhanced postoperative predictability and refractive accuracy as compared with conventional IOL power calculation formulae. At present, the outcomes with the new-generation IOL power calculation formulae such as Barrett Universal II are largely comparable to AI-based formulae. Incorporation of additional variables such as IOL design, larger datasets representative of different population groups, and sophisticated AI algorithms can help further enhance accuracy and move toward the goal of customized IOL power for each individual.

CONCLUSION

Artificial intelligence is increasingly being incorporated in IOL power calculation formulae to improve predictability. Machine-learning models based on neural network, SVR, and XGBoost are commonly employed to predict IOL power based on large datasets of outcomes. Commonly used AI-based formulae include Hill-RBF 3.0, Kane, Ladas Super Formula 2.0, PEARL-DGS, and Hoffer QST among others. The use of these formulae has improved the postoperative predictability and refractive accuracy, and the outcomes are comparable to newer generation IOL power calculation formulae such as Barrett Universal II. Limitations include unreliable results for eyes with unusual biometry, and the dataset may not be representative of different ethnicities.

REFERENCES

1. Kane JX, Van Heerden A, Atik A, Petsoglou C. Accuracy of 3 new methods for intraocular lens power selection. J Cataract Refract Surg. 2017;43:333-9.
2. Aristodemou P, Knox Cartwright NE, Sparrow JM, Johnston RL. Formula choice: Hoffer Q, Holladay 1, or SRK/T and refractive outcomes in 8108 eyes after cataract surgery with biometry by partial coherence interferometry. J Cataract Refract Surg. 2011;37:63-71.
3. Cooke DL, Cooke TL. Comparison of 9 intraocular lens power calculation formulas. J Cataract Refract Surg. 2016;42:1157-64.
4. Ladas J, Ladas D, Lin SR, Devgan U, Siddiqui AA, Jun AS. Improvement of multiple generations of intraocular lens calculation formulae with a novel approach using artificial intelligence. Transl Vis Sci Technol. 2021;10:7.
5. Mori Y, Yamauchi T, Tokuda S, Minami K, Tabuchi H, Miyata K. Machine learning adaptation of intraocular lens power calculation for a patient group. Eye Vis. 2021;8:42.
6. Sramka M, Slovak M, Tuckova J, Stodulka P. Improving clinical refractive results of cataract surgery by machine learning. PeerJ. 2019;7:e7202.
7. Carmona González D, Palomino Bautista C. Accuracy of a new intraocular lens power calculation method based on artificial intelligence. Eye Lond Engl. 2021;35:517-22.
8. Hill-RBF 3.0. IOL Power calculator for cataract surgery | Hill-RBF Calculator. [online] Available from https://rbfcalculator.com/ [Last accessed January, 2024].
9. Kane Formula. [online] Available from https://www.iolformula.com/agreement/ [Accessed January, 2024].
10. Ladas JG, Siddiqui AA, Devgan U, Jun AS. A 3-D "super surface" combining modern intraocular lens formulas to generate a "super formula" and maximize accuracy. JAMA Ophthalmol. 2015;133:1431-6.
11. Kenny PI, Kozhaya K, Truong P, Weikert MP, Wang L, Hill WE, et al. Efficacy of segmented axial length and artificial intelligence approaches to intraocular lens power calculation in short eyes. J Cataract Refract Surg. 2023;49:697-703.
12. Debellemanière G, Dubois M, Gauvin M, Wallerstein A, Brenner LF, Rampat R, et al. The PEARL-DGS formula: The development of an open-source machine learning-based thick IOL calculation formula. Am J Ophthalmol. 2021;232:58-69.
13. Taroni L, Hoffer KJ, Pellegrini M, Lupardi E, Savini G. Comparison of the new Hoffer QST

with 4 modern accurate formulas. J Cataract Refract Surg. 2023;49:378-84.
14. Darcy K, Gunn D, Tavassoli S, Sparrow J, Kane JX. Assessment of the accuracy of new and updated intraocular lens power calculation formulas in 10 930 eyes from the UK National Health Service. J Cataract Refract Surg. 2020;46:2-7.
15. Nemeth G, Kemeny-Beke A, Modis L. Comparison of accuracy of different intraocular lens power calculation methods using artificial intelligence. Eur J Ophthalmol. 2022; 32:235-41.
16. Li T, Stein J, Nallasamy N. AI-powered effective lens position prediction improves the accuracy of existing lens formulas. Br J Ophthalmol. 2022;106:1222-6.
17. Kothari SS, Reddy JC. Recent developments in the intraocular lens formulae: An update. Semin Ophthalmol. 2023;38: 143-50.
18. Wan KH, Lam TCH, Yu MCY, Chan TCY. Accuracy and precision of intraocular lens calculations using the new Hill-RBF version 2.0 in eyes with high axial myopia. Am J Ophthalmol. 2019;205:66-73.

SECTION 4

Intraocular Lens Power Calculation in Challenging Situations

10. Post-refractive Surgery Intraocular Lens Power Calculation
11. Intraocular Lens Power Calculation in Children
12. Intraocular Lens Power Calculation in Corneal Pathologies
13. Intraocular Lens Power Calculation in Posterior Segment Pathology
14. Intraocular Lens Power Calculation in Extremes of Axial Length
15. Intraocular Lens Power of Piggyback IOLs and Secondary IOLs

CHAPTER 10

Post-refractive Surgery Intraocular Lens Power Calculation

■ INTRODUCTION

The armamentarium of modern-day refractive surgery includes corneal ablative procedures, namely photorefractive keratectomy (PRK), laser-assisted in situ keratomileusis (LASIK), small incision lenticule extraction (SMILE), and phakic intraocular lens (pIOL) implantation. These patients subsequently present for cataract surgery, and accurate biometry and IOL power calculation is challenging especially in the absence of adequate preoperative data. Radial keratotomy (RK) is no longer the procedure of choice for refractive correction; however, patients who have undergone RK in 1970–90s present for cataract surgery and may be particularly challenging to manage.

Cornea-based refractive surgical procedures lead to an altered corneal curvature and shape, which impacts the accuracy of keratometry estimation and IOL power calculation. This is further compounded by the high expectations of this subset of patients having undergone refractive correction for spectacle independence, as they are usually desirous of spectacle independence after cataract surgery as well. In this chapter, we discuss the sources of error in IOL power calculation after prior refractive surgeries, the IOL power calculation formulae to be used in these scenarios, and IOL selection keeping in mind the patient expectations.

■ IOL POWER CALCULATION AFTER CORNEAL ABLATIVE PROCEDURES

Corneal ablative procedures including PRK and LASIK lead to an alteration in corneal curvature and shape, with an altered anterior to posterior corneal curvature ratio. Various formulas are available for accurate IOL power calculation, that may or may not rely on pre-refractive surgery refraction and keratometry.

Sources of Error in IOL Power Calculation

Error in IOL power calculation after corneal ablative procedures may be attributed to the use of standard keratometric index, limitations of keratometry devices, and the use of wrong formulae.

Keratometric Index Error

A standard keratometric index of 1.3375 is used by conventional keratometry devices to estimate the corneal power, based on the assumption of a constant anterior to posterior corneal curvature ratio.[1,2] Corneal ablative procedures lead to a change in the anterior corneal surface without a significant corresponding change in the posterior corneal surface, thus disrupting this constant ratio and invalidating the use of the effective keratometric index.

Myopic LASIK or PRK leads to selective anterior corneal flattening with increase in radius of curvature, and the use of the standard keratometric index leads to an overestimation of corneal power with underestimation of IOL power and postoperative hyperopia. The reverse is observed after hyperopic LASIK/PRK correction, with tendency toward postoperative myopic error.

Radius Error or Instrument Error

Conventional keratometers and corneal topographers measure the simulated keratometry in the paracentral region of 2–4 mm.[3] Corneal curvature in optical axis is not measured, with the paracentral measurements extrapolated to obtain the central power. Myopic corneal ablative procedures lead to central flattening, and the measured paracentral corneal curvature is steeper than the central cornea. This difference is exaggerated in cases with small or decentered optical zone and negligible in eyes with larger optical zones of >6 mm.

The formula used in keratometers to calculate the corneal power is valid only for a spherical surface. Post-myopic ablation corneas are oblate rather than prolate, with maximum flattening at the center and progressive steepening with the ablation zone.[4] The change in corneal asphericity induced by laser refractive surgery may also contribute to an error in IOL power calculation.

Formula Error

Third-generation formulae (SRK-T, Holladay 1, and Hoffer Q) use axial length (AL) and keratometry (K) to calculate the effective lens position (ELP). Myopic corneal ablation leads to corneal fattening with no significant change in the anterior chamber depth (ACD), and consequently the ELP.

The use of flatter post-myopic refractive surgery K for ACD estimation results in an underestimation of ELP and IOL power. The reverse is true in post-hyperopic corneal ablative procedures. Formulas such as Haigis, Shammas-PL, and Olsen C constant which do not calculate the ELP based on K are negligibly affected by this error.[5]

IOL Power Calculation Methods

Methods for IOL power calculation in post-corneal refractive surgery may be categorized based on those based on historical data alone, those based on preoperative historical data and postoperative keratometry, and those that do not require any historical data **(Flowchart 1)**.

IOL Power Calculation Methods based on 100% Historical Data

The IOL power calculation methods based on 100% historical data include the clinical history method, Feiz-Mannis IOL power adjustment, and corneal bypass method **(Table 1)**. The accuracy of these methods is dependent upon the availability of reliable preoperative data, which may not be feasible in all cases.

Clinical history method: Clinical history method was the gold standard for post-refractive surgery IOL power calculation for two decades since its introduction by Holladay in 1989 for post-RK eyes; subsequently, Hoffer described it for post-PRK and post-LASIK eyes.[6] Postoperative corneal power is derived by subtracting the surgically induced refractive change (SIRC) in the corneal plane from preoperative K. It is a simple method without the need for complex formulae or algorithms and assumes a 1:1 relation between corneal dioptric power and refraction; however, postsurgical change in

CHAPTER 10: Post-refractive Surgery Intraocular Lens Power Calculation

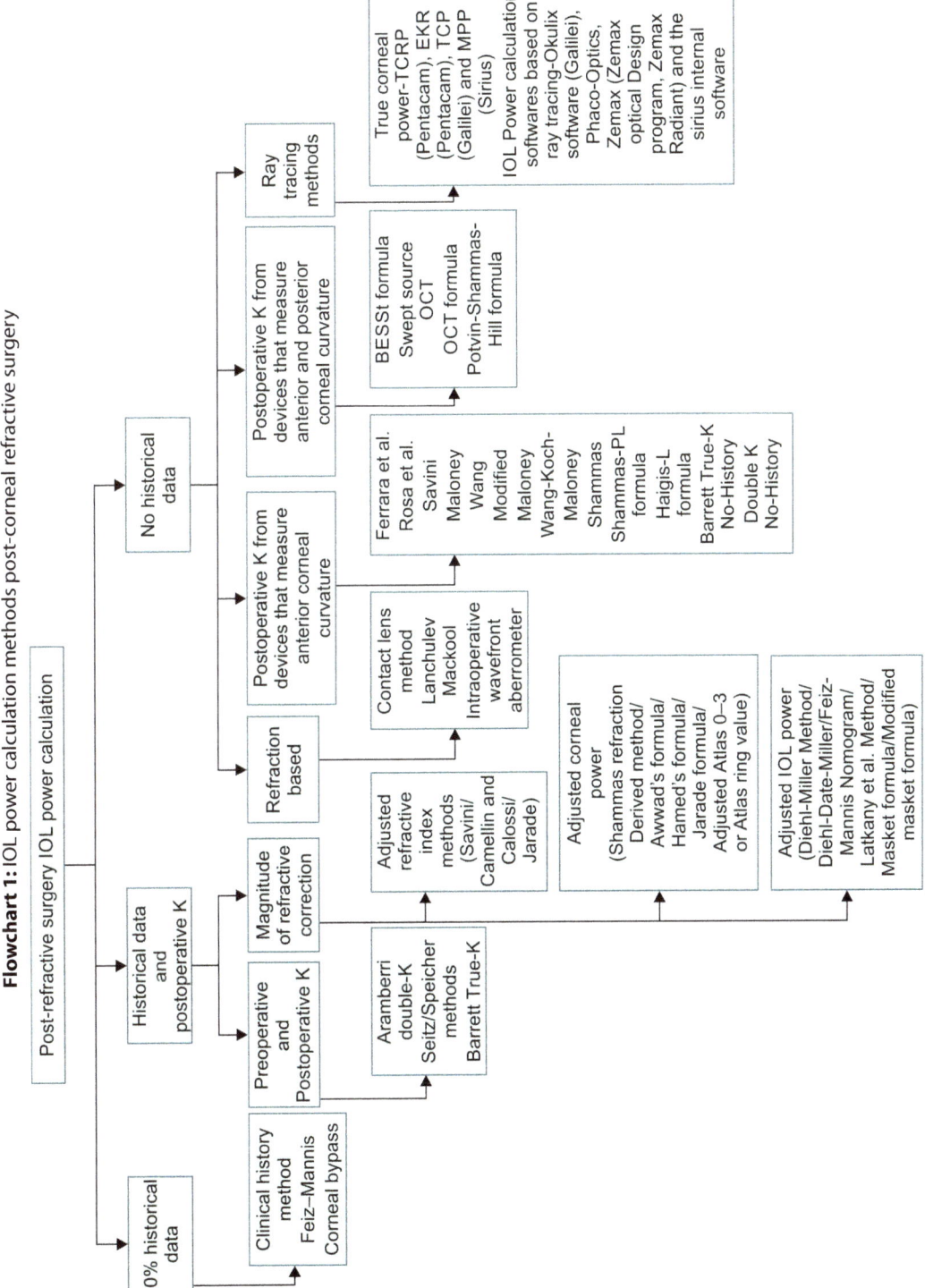

Flowchart 1: IOL power calculation methods post-corneal refractive surgery

TABLE 1: IOL power calculation methods based on 100% historical data

Method	Input variables	Formula	Output variable
Clinical history method	Preop K, SIRC	Kpost = Kpre − SIRC	Corrected K
Feiz Mannis IOL power adjustment method	Preop K change in SE	Corrected IOL power = IOL power using preop K + (ΔSE*0.7)	Corrected IOL power
Corneal bypass method	Preop K Net RE change	IOL power calculated using preop K; RE correction at spectacle plane used as target refraction • Corneal bypass or wake forest method—Holladay 1 • Ladas stark method—SRK/T	Corrected IOL power

(Preop: preoperative; K: keratometry; SIRC: surgically induced refractive change; Kpost: postoperative keratometry; Kpre: preoperative keratometry; IOL: intraocular lens; ΔSE: change in spherical equivalent; RE: refractive error)

corneal power is less (0.67–0.7 D per diopter refractive error) than the actual change in refraction.[7] SIRC at the spectacle plane is more accurate than SIRC at the corneal plane.[8]

Feiz–Mannis IOL power adjustment method:[9] The Feiz–Mannis method is based on the assumption that the difference between pre-LASIK and post-LASIK emmetropic IOL power should balance the change in spherical equivalent (SE). For every 1 D change in IOL power, the SE at spectacle plane changes by 0.7 D only, based on the IOL position behind the iris and a vertex distance of 12–13 mm.

Corneal bypass method: Corneal bypass method uses the refractive correction achieved by LASIK/PRK in the spectacle plane as the target refraction to select the IOL power. Preoperative keratometry is used to calculate the IOL power, and this method effectively bypasses the need for postoperative corneal power in IOL power calculation. The corneal bypass or Wake Forest method utilizes the Holladay I formula, whereas the Ladas-Stark method uses the SRK/T formula for IOL power calculation.[10,11]

Methods based on Historical Data and Postoperative Keratometry

These methods may be further subcategorized based on the input variables required including preoperative keratometry and SIRC.

Methods based on preoperative and postoperative keratometry:

- *Aramberri Double-K method:* Aramberri et al. suggested the use of both preoperative and postoperative keratometry for IOL power calculation.[5] Preoperative keratometry is used to estimate the ELP; the corrected postoperative keratometry obtained using the clinical history method is then used in the vergence formula to calculate final IOL power. It requires accurate preoperative data like K and SIRC, depending on the method to calculate corrected postoperative K.
- *Seitz/Speicher methods:*[2,4] The method is based on the assumption that total corneal power is the sum of anterior and posterior corneal surface powers, and the posterior corneal curvature does not change significantly after laser ablative surgery. Anterior corneal surface power may be calculated by multiplying the

measured keratometry value by 1.14 (0.376/0.3375). The total corneal power is calculated as the sum of postoperative anterior corneal power (Pa_{postop}) and preoperative posterior corneal power (P_{Ppreop}).
- *Barrett True-K formula:* It is a theoretical formula based on the Barrett Universal II,[12] and calculates the modified K based on the pre- and postrefractive surgery keratometry. It is incorporated in Lenstar 900 (Haag Streit, USA) and also available on ASCRS website (*www.ascrs.org*) and Asia-Pacific Association of Cataract and Refractive Surgeons website (*www.apacrs.org*).

Methods based on magnitude of refractive correction and postoperative keratometry: Magnitude of refractive correction (ΔMR) and postrefractive surgery keratometry have been used to calculate adjusted refractive index, adjusted keratometry, and corrected IOL power for patients undergoing cataract surgery.
- *Adjusted refractive index methods:* The standard keratometric index of 1.3375 is not accurate in post-refractive surgery eyes. Various methods adjust the index of refraction to accurately predict postoperative corneal power, including by Savini et al.,[13] Camellin and Calossi et al.,[14] and Jarade et al.,[15] as summarized in **Table 2**.[15] Postoperative corneal power (P_{Post}) can then be calculated using the equation $P_{Post} = (n_{post}-1)/r$, where, r is the measured postoperative anterior corneal curvature.

Good results have been observed using the Jarade method with Hoffer Q formula,[16] Camellin and Colossi method with Holladay formula (Double-K method), and Savini method with SRK-T formula (Double-K method).[17,18]

- *Adjusted keratometry based on SIRC and postoperative keratometry:* Adjusted keratometry values may be calculated by modifying the post-refractive surgery keratometry values based on the magnitude of refractive correction **(Table 2)**. Shammas refraction derived method,[19] Awwad's formulae,[20] Hamed's formula,[21] Jarade formula,[22] and Adjusted Atlas 0-3 or Atlas ring value[23] provide adjusted keratometry values, which may then be used with conventional IOL power calculation formulae (preferably Double-K modified methods).
- *Target refractive error calculation and IOL power adjustment:* Various methods and nomograms have been described to calculate the target refractive error based on ΔMR. Standard IOL power calculation formulae (Hoffer Q, Holladay 1, or SRK-T) may be used to calculate the IOL power with a target error derived from the formula **(Table 2)**.

Diehl-Miller[24] and Diehl-Date-Miller[25] nomograms describe a mathematical relationship between ΔMR and target refractive error to achieve emmetropia after cataract surgery. Diehl-Date-Miller used Pentacam K and 3rd generation formulae for IOL power calculation.[25] Feiz-Mannis nomogram used ΔMR at the spectacle plane.[8] Latkany et al.[26] observed flat K readings to be more accurate than average K, and adjusted the postoperative flatter K reading based on the pre-LASIK SE. Masket[27] suggested an adjustment for the calculated emmetropic IOL power where the SE of the total laser treatment (LSE) is used to calculate the corrective factor; the method was further modified by Hill et al. to give the modified Masket formula.

TABLE 2: IOL power calculation methods based on historical data and postoperative keratometry

Input variables	Output variable	Method	Calculations
Preoperative and postoperative keratometry	Corrected ELP and K	Aramberri Double-K	• Preop K—ELP estimation • Postop K—obtained using clinical history method • IOL power calculated using vergence formula to calculate final IOL power
	Corrected K	Seitz/Speicher methods	$P_{Postop} = SimK_{Postop} (1.14) + [SimK_{preop} - 1.14 \times SimK_{preop}]$
	Corrected IOL power	Barrett True-K	Formula incorporated in Lenstar 900; available with ASCRS online calculator (www.ascrs.org) and Asia-Pacific Association of Cataract and Refractive Surgeons website (www.apacrs.org)
Magnitude of refractive correction and postoperative keratometry	Adjusted refractive index	Savini et al. method	$n_{post} = 1.338 + 0.0009856 \times \Delta MR$
		Camellin and Calossi et al.	$n_{post} = 1:3319 + 0.00113 \times \Delta MR$ (spectacle plane) $n_{post} = 1:3375 + 0.0014 \times \Delta MR$ (corneal plane)
		Jarade et al.	
	Corrected K	Shammas refraction derived method	Corrected $K = K_{post} - 0.23 \times CRc$
		Awwad's formula	$ACCP_{adj} = ACCP - (\Delta MR \times 0.16)$
		Hamed's formula	Adjusted EffRP = (EffRP) $- 0.15 \times \Delta MR - 0.05$
		Jarade formula	$K_{postop} = K_{preop} - [(0.376) \times (R_{a-postop} - R_{a-preop})/(R_{a-postop} \times R_{a-preop})]$
		Adjusted Atlas 0–3 or Atlas ring value*	Adjusted Atlas 0–3 = (Atlas 0–3) $- 0.2 \times \Delta MR$
	Corrected IOL power	Diehl-Miller Method	Target error $= -0.018 (\Delta MR)^2 + 0.192 (\Delta MR) - 0.062$
		Diehl-Date-Miller	Target error $= -0.0198 (\Delta MR)^2 + 0.170 (\Delta MR) - 0.0079$
		Feiz-Mannis nomogram	• IOL power underestimation $= -0.231 + (0.595 \times \Delta MR)$ {For myopic LASIK} • IOL power overestimation $= 0.751 - (0.862 \times \Delta MR)$ {For hyperopic LASIK}
		Latkany et al. method	• Postmyopic LASIK/PRK—Adjusted $IOL_{flatK} = IOL_{flatK} - (0.47x + 0.85)$ • Using average K—Adjusted $IOL_{avgk} = IOL_{avgk} - (0.46x + 0.21)$ • Post-hyperopic LASIK—Adjusted $IOL_{flatk} = IOL_{flatk} - (0.27x + 1.53)$
		Masket formula	IOL power adjustment = LSE $\times (-0.326) + 0.101$
		Modified Masket formula	IOL power adjustment = LSE $\times (-0.4385) + 0.0295$

*Adjusted Atlas 9000 (4-mm zone) uses the average power over the 4 mm zone

[ΔMR: change in manifest refraction; ACCP: anterior central corneal power; ACCP$_{adj}$: final adjusted anterior central corneal power; CRc: myopic correction in corneal plane; EffRP: effective refractive power (obtained from the EyeSys corneal analysis system, EyeSys Vision, Inc.); ELP: effective lens position; IOL: intraocular lens; K: keratometry; K$_{post}$: postoperative keratometry; Kpre: preoperative keratometry; LSE: spherical equivalent of total laser correction; n$_{post}$: postoperative corrected refractive index; P$_{Postop}$: postoperative corneal power; Preop: preoperative; R$_{a-postop}$: postoperative radius of curvature; R$_{a-preop}$: preoperative radius of curvature; SimK$_{Postop}$: postoperative simulated keratometry; SimK$_{preop}$: preoperative simulated keratometry; SIRC: surgically induced refractive change; x: prerefractive surgery spherical equivalent (myopic or hyperopic)]

IOL Power Calculation Methods: No Historical Data

The IOL power calculation in the absence of historical data includes contact lens method, methods based on intraoperative aphakic refraction, modified formulae, and methods employing either the anterior corneal curvature measurements or both anterior and posterior corneal curvature, as well as ray tracing methods.

Refraction-based methods: Refraction-based methods include contact lens method, which is now obsolete, intraoperative aphakic refraction, and intraoperative aberrometry.

- *Contact lens method:* Contact lens (CL) method was originally described by Holladay in post-RK patients and mainly of historical interest.[28] The method is based on the determination of the difference between the manifest refraction with and without a hard contact lens (PMMA) of a known base curve. The method is obsolete now owing to poor accuracy and reliability in cataractous eyes.
- *Methods based on intraoperative aphakic refraction:* Methods based on aphakic refraction are not dependent on preoperative or postoperative biometry values or change in SE. However, surgery needs to be paused to perform refraction resulting in increased surgical time. Accuracy of intraoperative readings is dependent on good patient cooperation and maintenance of optimum IOP. Ianchulev et al.[29] and Mackool et al. proposed equations to calculate final adjusted IOL power based on the intraoperative aphakic refraction. Intraoperative wavefront aberrometer (Optiwave Refractive Analysis System, Alcon Laboratories, Inc., Fort Worth, Texas, USA) has been used to perform intraoperative refractive biometry for calculating IOL power.[30] IOL power is calculated based on aphakic SE and AL and K (measured before cataract surgery) to estimate the ELP. Optimal results have been demonstrated with this method, with better accuracy than Haigis-L and Shammas PL.

Methods using keratometry based on anterior corneal curvature measurements: Modifications of simulated keratometry values from standard keratometers, optical biometers, and central corneal power from corneal topographers have been described to enable accurate IOL power calculation **(Table 3)**. Ferrara et al.[31] proposed theoretical variable refractive index (TRI) based on AL; similarly, Rosa et al. proposed a regression formula to determine radius correcting factor (RCF) for different ALs. These were then used to calculate the corrected K.

- *Savini method*[31] is a modification of the Seitz/Speicher method to calculate postoperative true corneal power when the preoperative corneal power is not known. A mean value –4.98D for posterior corneal surface is used, and postoperative corneal power is derived from the equation:

$$P_{Postop} = SimK_{Postop} (1.14) - 4.98$$

- *Methods using central corneal power from Atlas topographer:* Various formulas and methods to derive corrected postoperative power use postoperative central corneal power from Atlas topographer rather than simulated keratometry (SimK) values, such as the *Maloney method, Wang method, Modified Maloney method,* and *Wang Koch Maloney method.* Maloney, Wang, and Modified Maloney use central corneal power from the Atlas topographer.

TABLE 3: IOL power calculation methods based on no historical data

Input variable	Output variable	Method	Calculations
Refraction	Corrected K	Contact lens method	True keratometry (K) = $B_{CL} + P_{CL} + R_{CL} - R_{NoCL}$
	Corrected IOL power	Ianchulev	Final adjusted IOL power = (2.10449 × intraoperative SE)
		Mackool	IOL Power = Aphakic Manifest Refraction SE × 1.75
		Intraoperative wavefront aberrometer	Proprietary formula based on aphakic SE, AL, and K
Postoperative keratometry (obtained from devices that measure anterior corneal curvature)	Corrected refractive index	Ferrara et al.	TRI = −0.0006 (AL × AL) + 0.0213 × AL + 1.1572 Corrected K_{Post} = (TRI − 1)/r
	Corrected K		
	Radius correcting factor	Rosa et al.	RCF = 0.0276 × AL + 0.3635 Corrected K_{Post} = (1.3375 − 1)/ [(R_{post} × RCF)/1,000]
	Corrected K	Savini	$P_{Postop} = SimK_{Postop}$ (1.14) − 4.98
		Maloney[#]	K = Central corneal power × 1.114 − 4.9
		Wang[#]	K = Central corneal power × 1.114 − 6.1
		Modified Maloney[#]	K = Central corneal power × 1.114 − 5.51
		Wang-Koch-Maloney[$]	K = Central corneal power × 1.114 − 5.59
		Shammas	Myopic ablation—K_{post} corrected = 1.14 K_{post} − 6.8 Hyperopic ablation—K_{post} corrected = 1.0457 K_{post} − 1.9538
	Corrected IOL power	Shammas-PL formula	C = (0.5835 × A) − 64.40 IOL power calculated using the measured axial length, corrected Km (Shammas method) and postoperative AC depth.
		Haigis-L[^] formula	$r_{corrected}$ = 0.3315/(−5.163 × measured radius of curvature + 82.260 − 0.35) Corrected radius of curvature used in Haigis formula
		Barrett True-K No-History	Internal regression formula
		Double-K No-History	Standard K of 43.6D used in ELP estimation instead of preoperative K Corrected ELP and K used in Holladay 1 formula

Contd...

Contd...

Input variable	Output variable	Method	Calculations
Postoperative keratometry (obtained from devices that measure both anterior and posterior corneal curvature)	Corrected K	BESSt formula	Corrected postoperative keratometric power calculated based on Pentacam K pachymetry (Oculus Pentacam) by modifying the Gaussian optics formula.
		Pentacam	EKR, TCRP, TNP
		Sirius tomographer	MPP
		Galilei tomographer	TCP
		Swept source OCT	Total keratometry
	Corrected IOL power	OCT formula	• ECP (post Myopic LASIK/PRK) = 1.0208 × net corneal power − 1.6622 • ECP (post-hyperopic LASIK/PRK) = 1.1 × net corneal power − 5.736 • IOL power calculated based on AL, ACD (from IOLMaster), posterior corneal power, net corneal power and the CCT (from OCT)
		Potvin-Shammas-Hill formula	Keratometric values obtained from the Pentacam TNP (4-mm zone) used in Shammas No-History formula
Ray tracing method	• True corneal power • True IOL power	Devices based on ray tracing principle	• True corneal power—TCRP (Pentacam), EKR (Pentacam), TCP (Galilei), and MPP (Sirius) • IOL Power calculation software based on ray tracing—Okulix software (Galilei), Phaco-optics, Zemax (Zemax optical Design Program, Zemax Radiant), and the Sirius internal software

Note:
#Central corneal power from Atlas topographer used
$Average power from the 4-mm zone of the Atlas topographer used as the central corneal power
^IOL Master K used
(A: A constant of the specific IOL; AL: axial length; B_{CL}: base curve of CL in Diopters; C: postoperative AC depth; ECP: effective corneal power; EKR: equivalent K readings; K: keratometry; MPP: mean pupil power P_{CL}: spherical power of the CL in Diopters; P_{Postop}: postoperative corneal power; RCF: radius correcting factor; R_{CL}: spherical equivalent refractive error with the contact lens at corneal plane; R_{NoCL}: spherical equivalent refractive error without the contact lens at corneal plane; SE: spherical equivalent; $SimK_{Postop}$: postoperative simulated keratometry; TCP: total corneal power; TCRP: total corneal refractive power; TNP: true net power; TRI: theoretical variable refractive index)

Wang Koch Maloney method uses the average power from the 4-mm zone of the Atlas topographer as the central corneal power. Maloney et al. method is recommended for use with SRK-T formula and Wang method[23] is recommended with Double-K Holladay 2 and Hoffer Q.

- *Shammas No-History method:*[32] Shammas et al. used keratometry value from a standard keratometer to calculate corrected postoperative keratometry after myopic ablation.[19]

$$K_{post}\ corrected = 1.14\ K_{post} - 6.8$$

For eyes post-hyperopic ablation, they proposed the following formula:[33]

$$K_{post}\ corrected = 1.0457\ K_{post} - 1.9538$$

- *Shammas-PL formula* is a post-LASIK modification of the Shammas formula, where final IOL power is calculated using the measured AL, corrected Km, and postoperative AC depth. Postoperative AC depth (C) is derived from the A-constant of the specific IOL, not the keratometry.

$$C = (0.5835 \times A) - 64.40$$

It is available on the ASCRS online calculator and incorporated in Lenstar 900 (Haag Streit, USA).

- *Haigis-L formula:* The Haigis-L formula essentially modified the keratometry value measured by the IOLMaster to be used in the standard Haigis formula. The formula is included in the operating software of the IOLMaster (version 4.0 and later, Carl Zeiss Meditec AG) and is available on the ASCRS online calculator. The algorithm is based on three concepts. First, corrected postoperative keratometry is calculated based on the postoperative keratometry obtained with IOLMaster using regression equation as follows:

$$K_{corrected} = -5.163 \times \text{measured radius of curvature} + 82.260$$

Next, a correction factor is subtracted from the calculated power to account for the ELP prediction error, as the measured ACD (which is measured from the corneal vertex) is shortened due to the ablative procedure

$$K_{corrected} = -5.163 \times \text{measured radius of curvature} + 82.260 - 0.35$$

This value is converted into radius of curvature using a keratometry index of 1.3315, as the Haigis formula requires K entry in radius of curvature and internally uses the 1.3315 conversion

$$r_{corrected} = 331.5/(-5.163 \times \text{measured radius of curvature} + 82.260 - 0.35)$$

Separate correction is applied for post-hyperopic LASIK eyes. Studies have reported accurate results using the formula.[34] The formula does not require any preoperative data and avoids the error in ELP prediction; however, IOLMaster and its keratometry reading is required.

- *Barrett True-K No-History method:* The Barrett True-K formula can be used even when the SE change history in unavailable. An internal regression formula calculates the change in manifest SE.[35]
- *Double-K No-History method:* The method is similar to the double-K method described earlier; average K value is entered instead of the actual preoperative K (43.86 D in the ASCRS online calculator).

Saiki et al.[36] proposed a modified double-K or the A-P method using the SRK-T formula, where postoperative posterior corneal curvature in 6-mm zone (Pentacam) was used to estimate the preoperative keratometry required for ELP estimation. The postoperative Km (from sagittal front map of Pentacam) was used in the vergence formula. Regression equation for estimated preoperative K is:

$$\text{Estimated Pre}_{Km} = -4.907 \times \text{Postop Posterior K} + 12.371$$

Methods using keratometry based on anterior and posterior corneal curvature measurements: Devices which measure both the anterior and posterior corneal surfaces provide total corneal power and help to increase the accuracy of post-keratorefractive surgery IOL power calculation.

- *BESSt formula:* The BESSt formula calculates corrected postoperative keratometric power taking into account the anterior and posterior corneal curvature and pachymetry (Oculus Pentacam) by modifying the Gaussian optics formula. It uses a variable rather than static index of refraction of each individual cornea based on CCT and measured anterior surface curvature. The corrected K was originally used in SRK-T and Hoffer Q formula (when AL <22 mm) with good results.[37]
- *Optical coherence tomography (OCT)-based methods:* Tang et al. proposed an OCT-based IOL calculation formula based on vergence tracing that would be unaffected by prior refractive surgery.[38] The OCT net corneal power obtained in virgin eyes was 1.2 D lower than that measured by conventional keratometry, and 2.89 D lower in post-LASIK eyes. The difference in these values predisposes to erroneous results with the direct use of OCT-based net corneal power in the standard formulas. OCT-based formula is a ray tracing formula based on optical vergence model of the eye. It uses five biometric parameters, namely AL, ACD (from IOLMaster), posterior corneal power, net corneal power, and the CCT (from OCT). Effective corneal power (ECP) based on linear regression analysis is calculated from net corneal power given by the equation:

    ECP (post-myopic LASIK/PRK) = 1.0208 × net corneal power − 1.6622

    ECP (post-hyperopic LASIK/PRK) = 1.1 × net corneal power − 5.736

    The results were comparable to Orbscan total K used in Holladay 2 formula (Double-K) and better than Haigis-L and Shammas-PL No-History formula.[39-41]
- *Swept source OCT (SS-OCT) and total keratometry (TK):* IOLMaster 700 (Carl Zeiss Meditec AG) uses a combination of telecentric keratometry and SS-OCT technology to assess the anterior and posterior corneal curvatures. TK is calculated based on the anterior corneal curvature, posterior corneal curvature, and corneal thickness and is compatible for use with the standard IOL formulae by applying the existing IOL constants. IOL power calculated using Haigis formula with the TK reading is very accurate and the outcomes are comparable to that obtained with Barrett True-K and Haigis-L formulas.[42]
- *Scheimpflug tomography for corneal power estimation:* Scheimpflug-based tomography devices can directly measure both the anterior and the posterior corneal surface including the geometrical center of the cornea. Three important devices employing the Scheimpflug imaging technology are Sirius (Costruzione Strumenti Oftalmici, Florence, Italy), Galilei (Ziemer Ophthalmic Systems AG, Port, Switzerland), and Pentacam HR (Oculus Optikgerate GmbH, Wetzlar, Germany).

- Pentacam provides equivalent K readings (EKR), true net power (TNP), and total corneal refractive power (TCRP).

  Equivalent K reading in Holladay EKR Detail Report calculates corneal power based on Snell's law, taking into account anterior surface, posterior surface, and corneal thickness and adding a correction factor to enable direct use in conventional IOL formula (which assume n = 1.3375). EKR within the 4- or 4.5-mm zone has been recommended for use in post-refractive surgery patients.[43]

  True net power is the sum of anterior and posterior corneal power calculated using a modified Gaussian optics formula. The direct use of TNP in the conventional IOL formulae is discouraged as it is based on paraxial approximation, leading to underestimation of corneal power.[43-45]

  Total corneal refractive power (TCRP) is determined using ray tracing without relying on the keratometric index of refraction. It is derived from the anterior and posterior corneal curvature, corneal thickness and refractive indices of aqueous humor, cornea and air using the Snell's Law. Studies have observed accurate outcomes with TCRP at varying zones, including 2-, 3-, and 4-mm zone.[46-48] TCRP at the 5-mm zone accurately reflects the SIRC after hyperopic corneal ablation.[49] TCRP is the most realistic corneal power depiction; however, it should not be directly used in conventional IOL formula, as calculation does not rely on paraxial optics. Seo et al.[50] proposed adding a conversion factor of 0.7D to correct underestimation of corneal power with TCRP, and the equivalent K thus obtained can be directly used in conventional IOL calculation formula such as Holladay 2.

- Galilei G6 combines partial coherence interferometry (PCI) optical biometer and dual Scheimpflug analyzer with placido disk. It calculates *total corneal power (TCP)* using ray tracing and the Gaussian equivalent power using Gaussian optics formula.[51] TCP values are lower than corneal power calculated using keratometric index in post-myopic LASIK and normal eyes, necessitating the need for appropriate formula-optimized constants when used in conventional formula.[52] TCP2 is used in ASCRS online calculator, and is the average total corneal power for the central 4-mm diameter of the cornea, calculated using the aqueous index of refraction (1.336) with the anterior corneal surface acting as the reference plane for the focal length determination.

- Sirius anterior segment evaluation system combines a rotating Scheimpflug camera with a placido disk topographer (Costruzione, Strumenti, Oftalmici, Florence, Italy) and can measure both the corneal surfaces directly. It provides *simulated keratometry (SimK)* and the *true net power (TNP)* based on Gaussian optics. The *mean pupil power (MPP)* is the mean corneal power calculated over the pupil by ray tracing. The $MPP_{4.5}$, MPP_5, and $MPP_{5.5}$ provide an accurate assessment of post-laser refractive surgery corneal power by closely mirroring the change in RE.[53]

- *Potvin-Shammas-Hill formula:* The *Potvin-Shammas-Hill formula* is used for IOL power calculation in post-LASIK patients and is available on the ASCRS online calculator. It is based on Shammas No-History formula and uses keratometric values obtained from the

Pentacam TNP (4-mm zone) instead of the clinically derived Kc described originally by Shammas.[54]

Ray Tracing

Ray tracing methods do not depend on preoperative data or empirical optimization for postoperative corneal power calculation.
- TCRP (Pentacam), TCP (Galilei), and MPP (Sirius) are corneal power measurements obtained using the ray tracing method. Corneal power obtained using ray tracing has been claimed to be the most accurate; however, some studies have reported slight underestimation or overestimation of corneal power values in normal and post-refractive surgery eyes.[43,55] It is important to customize or optimize the keratometry values obtained using ray tracing methods before using them in standard IOL calculation formulae.
- Alternatively, commercially available software with their own IOL position prediction algorithms allow IOL power calculation using these measurements directly. These include the Okulix software (Galilei), Phaco-Optics, Zemax (Zemax Optical Design Program, Zemax Radiant), and the Sirius internal software. A recent study reported IOL power calculation using the Okulix software in the GalileiG6 device and Barrett True-K method to be the most accurate in post-myopic LASIK/PRK patients with no historical data, with 63.6% of eyes being within 0.5D of target error.[56]

ASCRS Online Calculator

American Society of Cataract and Refractive Surgery (ASCRS) website has an online post-refractive surgery IOL calculator, designed in 2007, which is available free of cost to all surgeons.

Three modules are available for IOL power calculation based on the refractive surgical procedure, namely myopic LASIK/PRK, hyperopic LASIK/PRK, and RK **(Table 4)**.

Fourteen methods are available for post-myopic LASIK/PRK IOL power calculation (9 for post-hyperopic LASIK/PRK), using either historical data in the form of magnitude of refractive correction (ΔMR) or using no prior data. The corrected keratometry obtained by these methods is used in five IOL power formulae, namely the Double-K Holladay 1, Shammas-PL, Haigis-L, OCT-based formula, and Barrett True-K to give the corrected IOL power. Masket and modified Masket methods directly provide the corrected IOL power. Maximum, minimum, and average IOL power using all methods is also provided in addition to the power calculated by individual methods.[57,58]

At present, version 4.9 is being used. Older methods based on preoperative K and ΔMR, such as CHM, corneal bypass, and Feiz-Mannis, have been removed due to poor accuracy, with addition of newer methods such as OCT-based formula, Barrett True-K, and Potvin-Hill method.

Outcomes

Methods based on historical data may achieve 53–85% of eyes within 0.5 D of target postoperative refraction; the predictability decreases to 45–85% in absence of historical data **(Table 5)**. Among the history-based methods, those requiring preoperative keratometry data perform worse than those requiring preoperative SE.[57,59] In absence of clinical history, regression-based formula like Barrett True-K, Shammas-PL No-History method, and Haigis-L not relying on any historical data performs better than other

TABLE 4: ASCRS online calculator for prior myopic LASIK/PRK

Type of method	Method	Description	IOL formula used
Based on change in magnitude of refraction	Adjusted EffRP	Adjusted EffRP = EffRP + (RC × 0.162) − 0.279 EffRP (Holladay Diagnostic Summary of the EyeSys Corneal Analysis System) samples all points within the central 3-mm cornea and takes into account the Stiles-Crawford effect	Double-K Holladay 1
	Adjusted Atlas 9000 (4-mm zone)	Adjusted corneal power = Atlas 9000 4-mm zone − (RC × 0.2)	Shammas-PL
	Adjusted Atlas ring values	Post-LASIK/PRK adjusted corneal power = Atlas Ring Values − (RC × 0.2) Average corneal power obtained by averaging the 0 mm, 1 mm, 2 mm, and 3 mm ring values on the Atlas 9000 or the numerical view from the Atlas 992-995 series	Double-K Holladay 1
	Masket formula	Adjusted IOL Power = IOL_{post} + (RC × 0.326) + 0.101	−
	Modified-Masket	Adjusted IOL Power = IOL_{post} + (RC × 0.4385) + 0.0295	−
	Adjusted ACCP/ACP/APP	Adjusted corneal power = ACCP − (RC × 0.16) • ACCP is the average of the mean powers of the central Placido rings over the central 3.0 mm of the cornea (Tomey Topography Modeling System) • Magellan ACP and OPD-Scan III APP 3-mm manual value modified using the same formula as the ACCP	Double-K Holladay 1
	Barrett True-K	Theoretical formula	Barrett True-K
No prior data	Wang-Koch-Maloney	Adjusted corneal power = (Atlas 4-mm zone × 1.114) − 5.59 D	Shammas-PL
	Shammas	Adjusted corneal power = 1.14 × K_{post} − 6.8 K_{post}-average K value from the IOLMaster	Shammas-PL
	Haigis-L	r corr = 331.5/(−5.1625 × r meas + 82.2603 − 0.35)	Haigis-L
	Galilei	TCP2—represents the average total corneal power for the central 4-mm diameter of the cornea calculated using the ray tracing method	Double-K Holladay 1
	Potvin-Hill pentacam	Estimates the post-LASIK/PRK corneal power using regression analysis using the TNP_Apex_Zone40 value from the Pentacam, and axial length and ACD value	Shammas-PL
	OCT	• Net corneal power, posterior corneal power and central corneal thickness obtained from RTVue or RTVue-XR (Optovue Inc.) • Axial length and anterior chamber depth from IOLMaster	OCT-based
	Barrett True K No-History	Theoretical formula	Barrett True-K

(ACCP: average central corneal power; ASCRS: American Society of Cataract and Refractive Surgery; EffRP: effective refractive power; IOL_{post}: IOL power after ablative corneal refractive surgery; K: keratometry; K_{post}: postoperative keratometry; r corr: corrected corneal radius; r meas: corneal radius in mm measured by the IOLMaster; RC: refractive correction at corneal plane; TCP2: total corneal power 2; TNP: true net power)

TABLE 5: Refractive outcomes with commonly used intraocular lens (IOL) power calculation methods in post-laser refractive surgery patients

IOL power calculation method/formula	Author/year	% of eyes within 0.5 D of target error	Median absolute prediction error (D)
Barrett True-K No-History	Wang (2019)*	52.8%	0.44
	Savini (2018)	60%	0.45
	Abulafia (2016)	63.3%	0.41
	Wang (2015)	58.7%	0.42
Barrett True-K with history	Abulafia (2016)	67.2%	0.33
	Savini (2018)	60%	0.48
	Wang (2015)	67.9%	0.33
Haigis-L	Wang (2019)*	45.3%	0.53
	Abulafia (2016)	46.7%	0.62
	Helaly (2016)	20%	0.74
	Fram (2015) (no historical data patients subset)	69%	0.26
	Fram (2015) (historical data patients subset)	85%	0.21
	Wang (2015)	55.8%	0.39
	Ianchulev (2014)	48%	0.53
	Huang (2013)	46%	0.65
	Yang (2013)	40%	–
	Wang (2010)	60%	–
Shammas-PL No-History	Abulafia (2016)	50%	0.53
	Savini (2018)	36.4%	0.79
	Helaly (2016)	26%	0.54
	Wang (2015)	52.9%	0.48
	Savini (2015)—No historical data subset	83.3%	0.31
	Ianchulev (2014)	50%	0.51
	Huang (2013)	46%	0.62
	Yang (2013)	45%	–
	McKarthy (2011)	53.8%	–
OCT-based formula	Fram (2015) (no historical data patients subset)	72%	0.28
	Fram (2015) (historical data patients subset)	60%	0.39
	Wang (2015)	68.3%	0.35
	Huang (2013)	59%	0.49
	Tang (2010)	78%	

Contd…

Contd...

IOL power calculation method/formula	Author/year	% of eyes within 0.5 D of target error	Median absolute prediction error (D)
Intraoperative aberrometry	Fram (2015) (no historical data patients subset)	74%	0.29
	Fram (2015) (historical data patients subset)	75%	0.25
	Ianchulev (2014)	67%	0.35
	Canto (2013)*	39%	–
Masket formula	Savini (2018)	73.3%	0.32
	Abulafia (2016)	60.3%	0.32
	Fram (2015)	85%	0.21
	Wang (2015)	64.3%	0.32
	Savini (2015)#	72.2%	0.24
	McKarthy (2011)—With Hoffer Q formula	58.8%	–
	Wang (2010)	57%	–
Modified Masket method	Abulafia (2016)	53.4%	0.48
	Wang (2015)	60.7%	0.30
	Wang (2010)	67%	
Using ray tracing software	Savini (2018)—best focus/paraxial	63.6%/63.5%	0.31/0.42
	Savini (2014)	71.4%	0.25
	Saiki (2014)	41.7%	0.62

Note:
*Included post hyperopic LASIK and RK eyes along with myopic LASIK/PRK eyes.
#In group 3 in which only SIRC known
(LASIK: laser-assisted in situ keratomileusis; OCT: optical coherence tomography; PRK: photorefractive keratectomy; SIRC: surgically induced refractive change)

methods, as the ELP prediction does not rely on the corneal curvature measurement. Newer methods such as intraoperative aberrometry, OCT-based formulae, and ray tracing methods result in nearly 70% patients with less than 0.5D predictive error **(Table 4)**. Recent network meta-analyses have reported OCT formula,[60,61] Barrett True-K no-history,[60,61] Masket,[60] and ORA (Optiwave Refractive Analysis)[61] as most accurate for calculating IOL power post-myopic laser vision correction. In a network meta-analysis evaluating the various no-history methods, ORA, BESSt, and Seitz/Speicher/Savini (Double-K SRK/T) were observed to be most accurate.[62] Despite promising results, at present, there is no standard accepted device that can exactly measure and calculate the total corneal power after corneal refractive surgery. **Flowchart 1** shows the possible options for IOL power calculation based on the data available.

IOL POWER CALCULATION IN POST-SMILE PATIENTS

Refractive lenticule extraction is a relatively recent addition to the armamentarium of refractive surgery, and the patients presenting for cataract surgery after SMILE are expected to increase in the subsequent decades.

As in corneal ablative procedures, IOL power calculation post-SMILE is expected to be challenging. As of now, the experience of IOL power calculation post-SMILE is extremely limited, and the predictability of IOL power calculation methods devised for corneal ablative patients has to be adequately assessed after refractive lenticule extraction.[63,64]

Measurement of Corneal Curvature

Anterior corneal curvature after SMILE has a relatively steeper central 2-mm zone with flatter periphery as compared with LASIK, with better preserved corneal asphericity. TCRP (4 mm) on Pentacam accurately reflects the change in manifest refraction post SMILE and may be used for IOL power calculation.[48] Holladay EKR values measured using Pentacam at 4 mm, 4.5 mm, and 5 mm have been observed to correlate well with the CHM-derived keratometry.[65,66]

The TCRP is calculated using ray tracing method and may be more accurate than EKR values. Qian et al. observed TCRP (3 and 4 mm zone) with customization to most accurately reflect the SE change in SMILE patients.[67] The 6.0 mm $TCRP_{apex,zone}$ and $TCRP_{pupil,zone}$ also compare well with the CHM-derived keratometry; however, inclusion of areas beyond the optical zone of SMILE while estimating keratometry may induce IOL power calculation errors.[65] Wei et al. devised a formula based on regression analysis to calculate the corrected postoperative K from Pentacam mean K for use in IOL power calculation, which had good agreement with CHM-derived keratometry.[66]

Corrected Postop K = 1.057 × Postoperative K – 3.146

They also proposed a refraction-derived method, using the postoperative mean K value obtained with Pentacam:

Corrected Postop K = 3.268 – 0.264 × SE change + 0.927 × postoperative K

IOL Power Calculation Methods

There is paucity of data regarding IOL power calculation post-SMILE, with only two studies evaluating actual outcomes after cataract surgery.[63,64]

Ray tracing method has been observed to be the most accurate for IOL power calculation post-SMILE.[68,69] Luft et al. used ray tracing method as the benchmark standard, and compared formulas on ASCRS online calculator for IOL power calculation in post-SMILE eyes. They observed lowest mean prediction error with Masket formula; in addition, Barrett True-K, Barrett True-K no-history, and Potvin Hill formula had comparable predictability as ray tracing method.[69]

Lischke et al. compared the predictability of various formulae in 11 post-SMILE eyes undergoing cataract surgery, and observed the smallest mean absolute error with the ray tracing method, with 82% and 91% of eyes within 0.5 D and 1 D of target error, respectively.[64] Potvin-Hill formula was also observed to be fairly accurate with 45% eyes within 0.5 D and 73% within 1D of predicted error.[64]

IOL POWER CALCULATION POST-RADIAL KERATOTOMY

Radial keratotomy was a popular choice for refractive correction in 1970–90s, and many of these patients require cataract surgery. Accurate IOL power calculation in post-RK cases may be challenging; in addition, the radial corneal incisions also cause unique intraoperative incision-related complications.

Sources of Error in IOL Power Calculation

The sources of error in estimating the corneal power are similar to post-LASIK/PRK eyes, with a few salient distinctions. Besides challenges in keratometry estimation, post-RK eyes are also associated with long-term hyperopic shift in 20–50% of patients, post-cataract surgery corneal edema, diurnal changes in refraction and the irregular corneal astigmatism which may be difficult to measure.

Keratometric Index Error

Radial keratotomy employs a variable number of radial midperipheral corneal incisions to flatten the cornea and correct myopic refractive error. The incisions induce central flattening with midperipheral steepening. Unlike LASIK/PRK, there is a change in the anterior–posterior curvature ratio post-RK, with the posterior surface flattening being more pronounced than the anterior surface flattening post-surgery. This results in an increase in the keratometric index (as opposed to the decrease observed after myopic LASIK/PRK).[70]

Radius Error/Instrument Error

The optical zone (OZ) after RK is usually 3 mm or less; however, manual keratometers measure corneal power at 3.2 mm zone. The entire cornea is flattened after RK, which spreads the keratometry mires even more peripherally, further worsening the accuracy of measurement. The central flatter cornea is not measured; there is overestimation of keratometry with underestimation of IOL power and postoperative hyperopia.[2,6] The error increases with increase in number of RK incisions and decrease in diameter of optical zone.

Formula Error

Formula error is attributed to the use of erroneous keratometry values for ACD and ELP estimation.

IOL Power Calculation Methods

Keratometry should be assessed at multiple times during the day to account for diurnal variation, with selection of the flattest K for IOL power calculation.[71] In addition, it is recommended to aim for –0.5 to –1.5D of postoperative myopia in post-RK patients to counteract the long-term hyperopic shift.

Corneal Power Measurement

Use of preoperative history is often difficult in post-RK patients, as the primary surgery would have been performed 20–30 years ago.[72] Chen et al. suggested the use of the flatter K obtained using CHM and CL method, with a target refraction of –1.5D to reduce postoperative hyperopia.[73] Adjusting the measured K reading by subtracting 1 D from it has also been suggested.[74]

Corneal power measurement from more central area, such as Average Central Corneal Power (ACCP) or Effective Refractive Power (EffRP, Holladay diagnostic summary of the EyeSys Corneal Analysis System) provides more accurate estimate of keratometry in post-RK patients.[75,76] Awwad et al. reported that $ACCP_{3mm}$ provided the best estimate of corneal power in post-RK patients; values from larger ($ACCP_{4mm}$) and smaller zones ($ACCP_{1mm}$ and $ACCP_{2mm}$) tend to overestimate and underestimate the power respectively.[76] Packer et al. observed 80% of post-RK eyes within 0.5 D of emmetropia with Holladay 2 formula using EffRP from EyeSys topographer.[75]

Tomographic methods such as Scheimpflug technology, OCT-based methods, and slit-scanning methods which measure both the anterior and posterior curvature provide a more accurate estimate of the central corneal power. They can also measure the geometrical center of the cornea. Demill et al. observed superior results with using average central power (ACP) from Pentacam K rather than keratometry measured from 1–4-mm zone on Atlas topographer with Holladay (Double-K) formula.[77]

IOL Power Formulae

Various methods have been suggested to obtain accurate postoperative power, similar to post-LASIK/PRK.

Third-generation formulas, such as Hoffer Q and Haigis, and fourth-generation formula using central corneal powers with or without a Double-K adjustment have shown reasonable outcomes after RK.[71,78] Potvin-Hill algorithm for IOL power calculation in post-RK eyes is based on the keratometry data from Pentacam used in Double-K Holladay 1 formula.[79] Post-RK module of ASCRS online calculator incorporates seven methods that calculate IOL power using Double-K Holladay 1, OCT-based, or Barrett True-K formulae.

Predictability of post-RK IOL power calculation has increased with availability of historical data, with post-RK refraction being the most important historical parameter and Barret True-K (history) being the most accurate formula. Post-RK version of the Barrett True-K formula in the ASCRS calculator underwent an update in 2016 and included the true K (history), true K (partial history), and true K (no history).

Among the no-history methods, Barrett True-K[72,80] has good outcomes, with 49–69% of eyes within 0.5 D of predicted error. OCT-based formula[81] and Haigis[71,72] have acceptable outcomes; however, their accuracy (40–50% eyes within 0.5D) is less than in post-LASIK/PRK cases.

Intraoperative aberrometry in post-RK eyes is less promising than in post-LASIK/PRK,[30,82] with only 40% post-RK eyes (67–74% in post PRK/LASIK) achieving a final RE within 0.5 D.[80]

IOL POWER CALCULATION IN PHAKIC IOL PATIENTS

Posterior chamber phakic IOLs do not have any significant effect on AL measured using immersion ultrasound or optical biometry.[83-85]

Post-phakic IOL AL measurements were observed to be longer after implantation of iris-fixated phakic IOLs, with decrease in measured ACD.[86] AL measurements may be distorted in the presence of a silicone phakic IOL.[87]

Optical biometry is more accurate than ultrasonic methods, and third-generation IOL power calculation formulae are preferred for IOL power calculation.

Newer formulas like Haigis and Barrett Universal II take into account the measured ACD for the estimation of ELP, which may change after removal of pIOL. Amro et al. observed a significant decrease in the ACD (measured with IOLMaster) after pIOL implantation and derived a regression formula to calculate the pre-phakic IOL ACD.[88] The reduction in ACD did not significantly affect the IOL power calculation, even with the use of Haigis or Barrett formulas. In addition, there was no significant change in keratometry and AL measurements after Implantable Collamer Lens (ICL) implantation. Intraoperative automated refraction, intraoperative aberrometry, and ray tracing methods are feasible alternatives for IOL power calculation after phakic IOL implantation.[88]

CHOICE OF IOL

Monofocal aspheric IOL is preferred in majority of cases. Myopic corneal ablative procedures induce positive spherical aberrations, and IOLs with negative spherical aberrations are preferred. Hyperopic LASIK/PRK induces negative spherical aberrations and IOL with zero spherical aberration is preferred.[89]

Toric IOL may be implanted in cases with regular astigmatism in the central 3-mm cornea, provided the axis and magnitude of toricity is repeatable, stable, and regular.

Patients that have undergone refractive surgery are desirous of spectacle independence after cataract surgery as well, and multifocal IOLs and extended depth of focus IOLs are increasingly being implanted after LASIK/PRK. Minimal corneal higher order aberrations, regular ocular surface, and absence of irregular corneal astigmatism should be documented before planning premium IOLs in these patients. Adequate patient counseling is a must to explain the risk of residual refractive error as well as dysphotopsia and decrease in visual quality.

CONCLUSION

Accuracy of post-refractive surgery IOL power calculation has increased with the advent of newer formulae and sophisticated diagnostic devices that measure both the anterior and posterior corneal curvature. ASCRS online calculator incorporates most of the current methods and formulae, and the surgeon can compare the IOL power obtained by different methods to select the desired power. With increasing popularity of SMILE, the next few decades will witness increasing number of cataract patients with prior history of SMILE, and slight modifications of existing formulae may be required to achieve optimal outcomes.

CLINICAL CASE EXAMPLES

CASE 1

A 45-year-old patient who underwent myopic LASIK 10 years ago was scheduled for right eye cataract surgery. Pre-LASIK refractive error was –7 DS in both eyes. Preoperative keratometry was not known.

Pre-cataract surgery parameters (right eye):

Axial length (AL)	29.65
Anterior chamber depth (ACD)	3.4 mm
Lens thickness (LT)	4.28 mm
Whit-to-white (WTW)	11.6 mm
K1/K2 (IOLMaster 700)	38.4 D/39.74 D
TK1/TK2 (IOLMaster 700)	38.11 D/39.02 D

(K: keratometry; TK: total keratometry)

The appropriate values were entered into the ASCRS postrefractive IOL calculator available online with a –0.5 D target.
- Patient received a +14 D IOL.
- His postoperative UCDVA was 6/6.

CHAPTER 10: Post-refractive Surgery Intraocular Lens Power Calculation

IOL Calculator for Eyes with Prior Myopic LASIK/PRK
(Your data will not be saved. Please print a copy for your record.)

Please enter all data available and press "Calculate"

Doctor Name		Patient Name		Patient ID	
Eye	OD	IOL Model	ICB00	Target Ref (D)	-0.5

Pre-LASIK/PRK Data:

Refraction*	Sph(D) -7	Cyl(D)* 0	Vertex (If empty, 12.5 mm is used)	12.5
Keratometry	K1(D)	K2(D)		

Post-LASIK/PRK Data:

Refraction*§	Sph(D) 0	Cyl(D)* 0	Vertex(If empty, 12.5 mm will be used)	12.5
Topography	EyeSys EffRP	Tomey ACCP / Nidek#ACP/APP	Galilei TCP2	
Atlas Zone value	Atlas 9000 4mm zone		Pentacam TNP_Apex_4.0 mm Zone	
Atlas Ring Values	0mm	1mm	2mm	3mm
OCT (RTVue or Avanti XR)	Net Corneal Power	Posterior Corneal Power	Central Corneal Thickness	

Optical/Ultrasound Biometric Data:

Ks	K1(D) 38.4	K2(D) 39.74	Device Keratometric Index (n) 1.3375 1.332 Other	
	AL(mm) 29.65	ACD(mm) 3.4	Lens Thick (mm) 4.28	WTW (mm) 11.6
Lens Constants**	A-const(SRK/T) 119.3	SF(Holladay1)		
	Haigis a0 (If empty, converted value is used)	Haigis a1 (If empty, 0.4 is used)	Haigis a2 (If empty, 0.1 is used)	

*If entering "Sph(D)", you must enter a value for "Cyl(D)", even if it is zero.
§Most recent stable refraction prior to development of a cataract.
Magellan ACP or OPD-Scan III APP 3-mm manual value (personal communication Stephen D. Klyce, PhD).
**Enter any constants available; others will be calculated from those entered. If ultrasonic AL is entered, be sure to use your ultrasound lens constants. It is preferable to use optimized a0, a1, and a2 Haigis constants.

[Calculate]   [Reset Form]

IOL calculation formulas used: Double-K Holladay 1[1], Shammas-PL[2], Haigis-L[3], OCT-based[4], & Barrett True K[5]

Using ΔMR		Using no prior data	
[1]Adjusted EffRP	--	[2]Wang-Koch-Maloney	--
[2]Adjusted Atlas 9000 (4mm zone)	--	[2]Shammas	13.30 D
[1]Adjusted Atlas Ring Values	--	[3]Haigis-L	12.24 D
Masket Formula	12.09 D	[1]Galilei	--
Modified-Masket	12.74 D	[2]Potvin-Hill Pentacam	--
[1]Adjusted ACCP/ACP/APP	--	[4]OCT	--
[5]Barrett True K	13.54 D	[5]Barrett True K No History	13.47 D

Average IOL Power (All Available Formulas): 12.90 D
Min: 12.09 D
Max: 13.54 D

SECTION 4: Intraocular Lens Power Calculation in Challenging Situations

CASE 2

A 50-year-old patient who underwent RK for 27 years ago was scheduled for right eye cataract surgery. Pre-RK refractive error was −2.5 DS in both eyes. Preoperative keratometry was not known.

IOL Calculator for Eyes with Prior RK
(Your data will not be saved. Please print a copy for your record.)

Please enter all data available and press "Calculate"

Doctor Name	Patient Name	Patient ID
Eye OD	IOL Model ZCB00	Target Ref(D) −0.5

Pre-RK Data:

Refraction Sph(D) −2.5   Cyl(D) 0   Vertex (If empty, 12.5 mm will be used)

Post-RK Data:

Refraction Sph(D) 0   Cyl(D) 0   Vertex(mm)

Topography	EyeSys EffRP	Average Central Power*		
Atlas Ring Values	1mm	2mm	3mm	4mm
Pentacam	PWR_SF_Pupil_4.0 mm Zone**	CT_MIN**		

OCT (RTVue or Avanti XR) Net Corneal Power   Posterior Corneal Power   Central Corneal Thickness

Optical/Ultrasound Biometric Data:

Ks   K1(D) 31.60   K2(D) 34.30   Device Keratometric Index (n)*** ● 1.3375 ○ 1.332 ○ Other

AL(mm) 24.66   ACD(mm) 2.95   Lens Thick (mm) 4.74   WTW (mm) 12.2

Lens Constants*** A-cons (SRK/T) 119.3   SF (Holladay1)

*Not SimK values; average central corneal powers from other devices.
**PWR_SF_Pupil_4.0 mm Zone refers to the Pentacam Power Distribution display for the Sagittal Curvature (Front) Mean (Km) value at a 4.0 mm zone and centered on the pupil. Click on PWR_SF_Pupil_4.0 mm Zone to see this topographic display. CT_MIN is the minimum central corneal thickness in microns as displayed by the Pentacam.
***Enter the constant available; the other will be calculated. If ultrasonic AL is entered, be sure to use your ultrasonic lens constants.

[Calculate]   [Reset Form]

IOL calculation formulas used: Double-K Holladay 1[1], OCT-based[2], & Barrett True K[3]

[1]EyeSys EffRP	--
[1]Average Central Power (other)	--
[1]Atlas 1-4	--
[1]Pentacam	--
[1]IOLMaster/Lenstar	33.99 D
[2]OCT	--
[3]Barrett True K	30.63 D

Average IOL Power: 32.31 D
Min: 30.63 D
Max: 33.99 D

Pre-cataract surgery parameters (right eye):

Axial length (AL)	24.66
Anterior chamber depth (ACD)	2.95 mm
Lens thickness (LT)	4.74 mm
Whit-to-white (WTW)	12.2 mm
K1/K2 (IOLMaster 700)	31.60 D/34.30 D
TK1/TK2 (IOLMaster 700)	32.77 D/34.73 D

(K: keratometry; TK: total keratometry)

The appropriate values were entered into the ASCRS post-refractive IOL calculator available online with a –0.5 D target.
- IOL power calculated using Haigis formula using TK on IOLMaster 700 was 32.5 D.
- Patient received a 34 D IOL and his postoperative UCDVA was 6/9. BSCVA was 6/6 with an acceptance of +0.5 DS.

REFERENCES

1. Olsen T. On the calculation of power from curvature of the cornea. Br J Ophthalmol. 1986;70:152-4.
2. Seitz B, Langenbucher A. Intraocular lens calculations status after corneal refractive surgery. Curr Opin Ophthalmol. 2000;11:35-46.
3. Savini G, Calossi A, Camellin M, Carones F, Fantozzi M, Hoffer KJ. Corneal ray tracing versus simulated keratometry for estimating corneal power changes after excimer laser surgery. J Cataract Refract Surg. 2014;40:1109-15.
4. Speicher L. Intra-ocular lens calculation status after corneal refractive surgery. Curr Opin Ophthalmol. 2001;12:17-29.
5. Aramberri J. Intraocular lens power calculation after corneal refractive surgery: double-K method. J Cataract Refract Surg. 2003;29:2063-8.
6. Hoffer KJ. Intraocular lens power calculation for eyes after refractive keratotomy. J Refract Surg. 1995;11:490-3.
7. Patel S, Alio JL, Perez-Santonja JJ. A model to explain the difference between changes in refraction and central ocular surface power after laser in situ keratomileusis. J Refract Surg. 2000;16:330-5.
8. Feiz V, Moshirfar M, Mannis MJ, Reilly CD, Garcia-Ferrer F, Caspar JJ, et al. Nomogram-based intraocular lens power adjustment after myopic photorefractive keratectomy and LASIK: a new approach. Ophthalmology. 2005;112:1381-7.
9. Feiz V, Mannis MJ, Garcia-Ferrer F, Kandavel G, Darlington JK, Kim E, et al. Intraocular lens power calculation after laser in situ keratomileusis for myopia and hyperopia: a standardized approach. Cornea. 2001;20:792-7.
10. Walter KA, Gagnon MR, Hoopes PC, Dickinson PJ. Accurate intraocular lens power calculation after myopic laser in situ keratomileusis, bypassing corneal power. J Cataract Refract Surg. 2006;32:425-9.
11. Ladas JG, Stark WJ. Calculating IOL power after refractive surgery. J Cataract Refract Surg. 2004;30:2458; author reply 2458-2459.
12. Barrett GD. An improved universal theoretical formula for intraocular lens power prediction. J Cataract Refract Surg. 1993;19:713-20.
13. Savini G, Barboni P, Zanini M. Correlation between attempted correction and keratometric refractive index of the cornea after myopic excimer laser surgery. J Refract Surg. 2007;23:461-6.
14. Camellin M, Calossi A. A new formula for intraocular lens power calculation after refractive corneal surgery. J Refract Surg. 2006;22:187-99.
15. Jarade EF, Abi Nader FC, Tabbara KF. Intraocular lens power calculation following LASIK: determination of the new effective index of refraction. J Refract Surg. 2006;22:75-80.
16. Kang BS, Han JM, Oh JY, Kim MK, Wee WR. Intraocular Lens Power Calculation after Refractive Surgery: A Comparative Analysis of Accuracy and Predictability. Korean J Ophthalmol. 2017;31:479-88.
17. Savini G, Barboni P, Carbonelli M, Ducoli P, Hoffer KJ. Intraocular lens power calculation after myopic excimer laser surgery: Selecting

the best method using available clinical data. J Cataract Refract Surg. 2015;41:1880-8.
18. Savini G, Hoffer KJ, Carbonelli M, Barboni P. Intraocular lens power calculation after myopic excimer laser surgery: clinical comparison of published methods. J Cataract Refract Surg. 2010;36:1455-65.
19. Shammas HJ, Shammas MC, Garabet A, Kim JH, Shammas A, LaBree L. Correcting the corneal power measurements for intraocular lens power calculations after myopic laser in situ keratomileusis. Am J Ophthalmol. 2003;136:426-32.
20. Awwad ST, Manasseh C, Bowman RW, Cavanagh HD, Verity S, Mootha V, et al. Intraocular lens power calculation after myopic laser in situ keratomileusis: Estimating the corneal refractive power. J Cataract Refract Surg. 2008;34:1070-6.
21. Hamed AM, Wang L, Misra M, Koch DD. A comparative analysis of five methods of determining corneal refractive power in eyes that have undergone myopic laser in situ keratomileusis. Ophthalmology. 2002;109:651-8.
22. Jarade EF, Tabbara KF. New formula for calculating intraocular lens power after laser in situ keratomileusis. J Cataract Refract Surg. 2004;30:1711-5.
23. Wang L, Booth MA, Koch DD. Comparison of intraocular lens power calculation methods in eyes that have undergone LASIK. Ophthalmology. 2004;111:1825-31.
24. Diehl JW, Yu F, Olson MD, Moral JN, Miller KM. Intraocular lens power adjustment nomogram after laser in situ keratomileusis. J Cataract Refract Surg. 2009;35:1587-90.
25. Date RC, Yu F, Miller KM. Confirmation and refinement of the Diehl-Miller nomogram for intraocular lens power calculation after laser in situ keratomileusis. J Cataract Refract Surg. 2013;39:745-51.
26. Latkany RA, Chokshi AR, Speaker MG, Abramson J, Soloway BD, Yu G. Intraocular lens calculations after retractive surgery. J Cataract Refract Surg. 2005;31:562-70.
27. Masket S, Masket SE. Simple regression formula for intraocular lens power adjustment in eyes requiring cataract surgery after excimer laser photoablation. J Cataract Refract Surg. 2006;32:430-4.
28. Haigis W. Corneal power after refractive surgery for myopia: contact lens method. J Cataract Refract Surg. 2003;29:1397-411.
29. Ianchulev T, Salz J, Hoffer K, Albini T, Hsu H, Labree L. Intraoperative optical refractive biometry for intraocular lens power estimation without axial length and keratometry measurements. J Cataract Refract Surg. 2005;31:1530-6.
30. Ianchulev T, Hoffer KJ, Yoo SH, Chang DF, Breen M, Padrick T, et al. Intraoperative refractive biometry for predicting intraocular lens power calculation after prior myopic refractive surgery. Ophthalmology. 2014;121: 56-60.
31. Savini G, Barboni P, Zanini M. Intraocular lens power calculation after myopic refractive surgery: theoretical comparison of different methods. Ophthalmology. 2006;113:1271-82.
32. Shammas HJ, Shammas MC. No-history method of intraocular lens power calculation for cataract surgery after myopic laser in situ keratomileusis. J Cataract Refract Surg. 2007;33:31-6.
33. Shammas HJ, Shammas MC, Hill WE. Intraocular lens power calculation in eyes with previous hyperopic laser in situ keratomileusis. J Cataract Refract Surg. 2013; 39:739-44.
34. Wang L, Tang M, Huang D, Weikert MP, Koch DD. Comparison of newer intraocular lens power calculation methods for eyes after corneal refractive surgery. Ophthalmology. 2015;122:2443-9.
35. Abulafia A, Hill WE, Koch DD, Wang L, Barrett GD. Accuracy of the Barrett True-K formula for intraocular lens power prediction after laser in situ keratomileusis or photorefractive keratectomy for myopia. J Cataract Refract Surg. 2016;42:363-9.
36. Saiki M, Negishi K, Kato N, Ogino R, Arai H, Toda I, et al. Modified double K method for intraocular lens power calculation after excimer laser corneal refractive surgery. J Cataract Refract Surg. 2013;39:556-62.
37. Borasio E, Stevens J, Smith GT. Estimation of true corneal power after keratorefractive

surgery in eyes requiring cataract surgery: BESSt formula. J Cataract Refract Surg. 2006; 32:2004-14.
38. Tang M, Li Y, Huang D. An intraocular lens power calculation formula based on optical coherence tomography: a pilot study. J Refract Surg. 2010;26:430-7.
39. Huang D, Tang M, Wang L, Zhang X, Armour RL, Gattey DM, et al. Optical coherence tomography-based corneal power measurement and intraocular lens power calculation following laser vision correction (an American Ophthalmological Society thesis). Trans Am Ophthalmol Soc. 2013;111: 34-45.
40. Tang M, Wang L, Koch DD, Li Y, Huang D. Intraocular lens power calculation after previous myopic laser vision correction based on corneal power measured by Fourier-domain optical coherence tomography. J Cataract Refract Surg. 2012;38:589-94.
41. Tang M, Wang L, Koch DD, Li Y, Huang D. Intraocular lens power calculation after myopic and hyperopic laser vision correction using optical coherence tomography. Saudi J Ophthalmol. 2012;26:19-24.
42. Wang L, Spektor T, de Souza RG, Koch DD. Evaluation of total keratometry and its accuracy for intraocular lens power calculation in eyes after corneal refractive surgery. J Cataract Refract Surg. 2019;45: 1416-21.
43. Ng ALK, Chan TCY, Cheng ACK. Comparison of Different Corneal Power Readings From Pentacam in Post-laser In Situ Keratomileusis Eyes. Eye Contact Lens. 2018;44(Suppl 2): S370-5.
44. Savini G, Barboni P, Profazio V, Zanini M, Hoffer KJ. Corneal power measurements with the Pentacam Scheimpflug camera after myopic excimer laser surgery. J Cataract Refract Surg. 2008;34:809-13.
45. Falavarjani KG, Hashemi M, Joshaghani M, Azadi P, Ghaempanah MJ, Aghai GH. Determining corneal power using Pentacam after myopic photorefractive keratectomy. Clin Exp Ophthalmol. 2010;38:341-5.
46. Savini G, Hoffer KJ, Carbonelli M, Barboni P. Scheimpflug analysis of corneal power changes after myopic excimer laser surgery. J Cataract Refract Surg. 2013;39:605-10.
47. Oh J-H, Kim SH, Chuck RS, Park CY. Evaluation of the Pentacam ray tracing method for the measurement of central corneal power after myopic photorefractive keratectomy. Cornea. 2014;33:261-5.
48. Gyldenkerne A, Ivarsen A, Hjortdal JØ. Assessing the corneal power change after refractive surgery using Scheimpflug imaging. Ophthalmic Physiol Opt. 2015;35: 299-307.
49. Whang W-J, Yoo Y-S, Joo C-K. Corneal power changes with Scheimpflug rotating camera after hyperopic LASIK. Medicine (Baltimore). 2018;97:e13306.
50. Seo KY, Im CY, Yang H, Kim TI, Kim EK, Kim T, et al. New equivalent keratometry reading calculation with a rotating Scheimpflug camera for intraocular lens power calculation after myopic corneal surgery. J Cataract Refract Surg. 2014;40:1834-42.
51. Wang L, Mahmoud AM, Anderson BL, Koch DD, Roberts CJ. Total corneal power estimation: ray tracing method versus gaussian optics formula. Invest Ophthalmol Vis Sci. 2011;52:1716-22.
52. Savini G, Negishi K, Hoffer KJ, Schiano Lomoriello D. Refractive outcomes of intraocular lens power calculation using different corneal power measurements with a new optical biometer. J Cataract Refract Surg. 2018;44:701-8.
53. Pan C, Hua Y, Huang J, Tan W, Lu W, Wang Q. Corneal Power Measurement With the Dual Scheimpflug-Placido Topographer After Myopic Excimer Laser Surgery. J Refract Surg. 2016;32:182-6.
54. Potvin R, Hill W. New algorithm for intraocular lens power calculations after myopic laser in situ keratomileusis based on rotating Scheimpflug camera data. J Cataract Refract Surg. 2015;41:339-47.
55. Savini G, Barboni P, Carbonelli M, Hoffer KJ. Accuracy of corneal power measurements by a new Scheimpflug camera combined with Placido-disk corneal topography for intraocular lens power calculation in

unoperated eyes. J Cataract Refract Surg. 2012;38:787-92.
56. Savini G, Hoffer KJ, Schiano-Lomoriello D, Barboni P. Intraocular lens power calculation using a Placido disk-Scheimpflug tomographer in eyes that had previous myopic corneal excimer laser surgery. J Cataract Refract Surg. 2018;44:935-41.
57. Wang L, Hill WE, Koch DD. Evaluation of intraocular lens power prediction methods using the American Society of Cataract and Refractive Surgeons Post-Keratorefractive Intraocular Lens Power Calculator. J Cataract Refract Surg. 2010;36:1466-73.
58. Yang R, Yeh A, George MR, Rahman M, Boerman H, Wang M. Comparison of intraocular lens power calculation methods after myopic laser refractive surgery without previous refractive surgery data. J Cataract Refract Surg. 2013;39:1327-35.
59. Chen X, Yuan F, Wu L. Metaanalysis of intraocular lens power calculation after laser refractive surgery in myopic eyes. J Cataract Refract Surg. 2016;42:163-70.
60. Pan X, Wang Y, Li Z, Ye Z. Intraocular lens power calculation in eyes after myopic laser refractive surgery and radial keratotomy: Bayesian network meta-analysis. Am J Ophthalmol. 2023:S0002-9394(23)00420-8. Online ahead of print.
61. Wei L, Meng J, Qi J, Lu Y, Zhu X. Comparisons of intraocular lens power calculation methods for eyes with previous myopic laser refractive surgery: Bayesian network meta-analysis. J Cataract Refract Surg. 2021; 47:1011-8.
62. Wen D, Yu J, Zeng Z, McAlinden C, Hu L, Feng K, et al. Network meta-analysis of no-History methods to calculate intraocular lens power in eyes with previous myopic laser refractive surgery. J Refract Surg. 2020; 36:481-90.
63. Ganesh S, Brar S, Sriprakash K. Post-small incision lenticule extraction phacoemulsification with multifocal IOL implantation: A case report. Indian J Ophthalmol. 2019; 67:1353-6.
64. Lischke R, Sekundo W, Wiltfang R, Bechmann M, Kreutzer TC, Priglinger SG, et al. IOL Power Calculations and Cataract Surgery in Eyes with Previous Small Incision Lenticule Extraction. J Clin Med. 2022;11:4418.
65. Pan C, Tan W, Hua Y, Lei X. Corneal power measurement with a new aberrometer/corneal topographer in eyes after small incision lenticule extraction for myopia. Int Ophthalmol. 2019;39:2815-24.
66. Wei P, Wang Y, Chan TCY, Ng ALK, Cheng GPM, Jhanji V. Determining total corneal power after small-incision lenticule extraction in myopic eyes. J Cataract Refract Surg. 2017; 43:1450-7.
67. Qian Y, Liu Y, Zhou X, Naidu RK. Comparison of Corneal Power and Astigmatism between Simulated Keratometry, True Net Power, and Total Corneal Refractive Power before and after SMILE Surgery. J Ophthalmol. 2017;2017:9659481.
68. Lazaridis A, Schraml F, Preußner P-R, Sekundo W. Predictability of intraocular lens power calculation after small-incision lenticule extraction for myopia. J Cataract Refract Surg. 2021;47:304-10.
69. Luft N, Siedlecki J, Schworm B, Kreutzer TC, Mayer WJ, Priglinger SG, et al. Intraocular Lens Power Calculation after Small Incision Lenticule Extraction. Sci Rep. 2020;10:5982.
70. Camellin M, Savini G, Hoffer KJ, Carbonelli M, Barboni P. Scheimpflug camera measurement of anterior and posterior corneal curvature in eyes with previous radial keratotomy. J Refract Surg. 2012;28:275-9.
71. Geggel HS. Intraocular Lens Power Selection after Radial Keratotomy: Topography, Manual, and IOLMaster Keratometry Results Using Haigis Formulas. Ophthalmology. 2015;122:897-902.
72. Turnbull AMJ, Crawford GJ, Barrett GD. Methods for Intraocular Lens Power Calculation in Cataract Surgery after Radial Keratotomy. Ophthalmology. 2020;127:45-51.
73. Chen L, Mannis MJ, Salz JJ, Garcia-Ferrer FJ, Ge J. Analysis of intraocular lens power calculation in post-radial keratotomy eyes. J Cataract Refract Surg. 2003;29:65-70.
74. Lyle WA, Jin GJ. Intraocular lens power prediction in patients who undergo cataract

surgery following previous radial keratotomy. Arch Ophthalmol. 1997;115:457-61.
75. Packer M, Brown LK, Hoffman RS, Fine IH. Intraocular lens power calculation after incisional and thermal keratorefractive surgery. J Cataract Refract Surg. 2004;30: 1430-4.
76. Awwad ST, Dwarakanathan S, Bowman RW, Cavanagh HD, Verity SM, Mootha VV, et al. Intraocular lens power calculation after radial keratotomy: estimating the refractive corneal power. J Cataract Refract Surg. 2007; 33: 1045-50.
77. DeMill DL, Moshirfar M, Neuffer MC, Hsu M, Sikder S. A Comparison of the American Society of Cataract and Refractive Surgery post-myopic LASI K/PRK Intraocular Lens (IOL) calculator and the Ocular MD IOL calculator. Clin Ophthalmol. 2011;5: 1409-14.
78. Stakheev AA, Balashevich LJ. Corneal power determination after previous corneal refractive surgery for intraocular lens calculation. Cornea. 2003;22:214-20.
79. Potvin R, Hill W. New algorithm for post-radial keratotomy intraocular lens power calculations based on rotating Scheimpflug camera data. J Cataract Refract Surg. 2013; 39:358-65.
80. Curado SX, Hida WT, Vilar CMC, Ordones VL, Chaves MAP, Tzelikis PF. Intraoperative Aberrometry Versus Preoperative Biometry for IOL Power Selection After Radial Keratotomy: A Prospective Study. J Refract Surg. 2019;35:656-61.
81. Ma JX, Tang M, Wang L, Weikert MP, Huang D, Koch DD. Comparison of Newer IOL Power Calculation Methods for Eyes With Previous Radial Keratotomy. Invest Ophthalmol Vis Sci. 2016;57:OCT162-8.
82. Fram NR, Masket S, Wang L. Comparison of Intraoperative Aberrometry, OCT-Based IOL Formula, Haigis-L, and Masket Formulae for IOL Power Calculation after Laser Vision Correction. Ophthalmology. 2015;122:1096-101.
83. Pitault G, Leboeuf C, Leroux les Jardins S, Auclin F, Chong-Sit D, Baudouin C. Optical biometry of eyes corrected by phakic intraocular lenses. J Fr Ophtalmol. 2005;28: 1052-7.
84. Khokhar SK, Agarwal T, Dave V. Comparison of preoperative and postoperative axial length measurement with immersion A-scan in ICL cases. J Cataract Refract Surg. 2009;35:2168-9.
85. Sanders DR, Bernitsky DA, Harton PJ, Rivera RR. The Visian myopic implantable collamer lens does not significantly affect axial length measurement with the IOLMaster. J Refract Surg. 2008;24:957-9.
86. Shin JY, Lee JB, Seo KY, Kim EK, Kim TI. Comparison of Preoperative and Postoperative Ocular Biometry in Eyes with Phakic Intraocular Lens Implantations. Yonsei Med J. 2013;54:1259-65.
87. Chen L-J, Chang Y-J, Kuo JC, Rajagopal R, Azar DT. Metaanalysis of cataract development after phakic intraocular lens surgery. J Cataract Refract Surg. 2008;34:1181-200.
88. Amro M, Chanbour W, Arej N, Jarade E. Third- and fourth-generation formulas for intraocular lens power calculation before and after phakic intraocular lens insertion in high myopia. J Cataract Refract Surg. 2018;44:1321-5.
89. Wang L, Koch DD. Intraocular Lens Power Calculations in Eyes with Previous Corneal Refractive Surgery: Review and Expert Opinion. Ophthalmology. 2021;128:e121-31.

Intraocular Lens Power Calculation in Children

CHAPTER 11

INTRODUCTION

Management of pediatric cataract is more challenging owing to delay in presentation or diagnosis, need for general anesthesia and postoperative visual rehabilitation including management of amblyopia. Intraocular lens (IOL) power remains a challenge in children, as the unpredictable growth pattern after surgery may adversely affect the refractive outcomes. Moreover, the conventional IOL formulae were originally developed for adult eyes and are less accurate in children. In younger children who are not cooperative for examination, the smaller eye and difficulty in performing an accurate biometry pose further challenges. Moreover, other factors such as the laterality of cataract, age at presentation, and refractive error in fellow eye need to be taken into consideration while choosing the IOL power. In this chapter, we highlight the various challenges in planning IOL implantation in a child and the recommended approaches to calculate the appropriate IOL power.

NORMAL DEVELOPMENT OF THE HUMAN EYE

The normal human eye undergoes axial length (AL) elongation, corneal flattening, and reduction in crystalline lens power during its growth from birth to adulthood. The gradual change in these three components contributes to the complex process of "emmetropization."

The AL exhibits a triphasic growth from birth to adulthood, increasing from a mean value of 16.8 mm at birth to 23.6 mm. The maximum growth occurs in the first 2 years, following which the rate decreases to about 0.4 mm/year till 5–6 years of age. It then increases by about 1 mm until adulthood. The keratometry values decrease from about 51.2 D at birth to 43.5 D in adulthood, with maximum change seen in the first 6 months of life. The mean crystalline lens power decreases from 34.4 D at birth to 18.8 D in adulthood, with the major reduction (of about 10 D) occurring in the first year of life.[1] In a child undergoing cataract surgery, the removal of lens results in a static lens power (aphakic or pseudophakic). The normal growth or increase in AL results in the increasing postoperative myopic shift or decrease in hyperopia.

REFRACTIVE GROWTH IN PSEUDOPHAKIC AND APHAKIC PEDIATRIC EYES

The growth of the eye in pediatric patients undergoing cataract surgery is highly variable, being affected by genetic and environmental factors that are incompletely understood.[2] While it is well established that the growth of the eye continues after cataract surgery wherein the rate is maximum during the first 2 years of age, it may continue beyond 10 years of age.[3] Accurate prediction of the AL growth and the accompanying refractive change after pediatric cataract surgery remains a challenge and is crucial to the selection of the appropriate IOL power in these patients.

Studies evaluating the refractive growth in pseudophakic and aphakic pediatric eyes have reported varying degrees of myopic shift post-surgery. An aphakic and pseudophakic eye shows an average myopic shift of 10 D and 5–7 D, respectively, from infancy to adulthood and follows a logarithmic curve. The shift is, however, highly variable with younger age at surgery consistently associated with greater and more unpredictable myopic shift.[4-6] The optical effect of the IOL can also contribute to the myopic shift observed. The fixed position of the IOL and elongation of the posterior segment relative to the anterior segment magnifies the myopic shift. The effective myopic shift is thus higher in eyes undergoing implantation of a higher power IOL due to this optical phenomenon, which is analogous to the effect of vertex distance.[2]

There is no correlation between the postoperative myopic shift and the initial AL or refractive target. Some studies have observed a higher myopic shift in children undergoing surgery for unilateral cataract surgery particularly in infancy, while others reported no difference between unilateral and bilateral cases.[7-9] The Infant Aphakia Treatment Study (IATS) reported that development of glaucoma and secondary visual axis opacity resulted in greater axial elongation.[10]

BIOMETRY

Children are often uncooperative for examination and lack precise fixation when examined under anesthesia.[11] Incorrect biometry, especially an AL measurement error, can produce a significant error in the calculated IOL power. A 1-mm error in AL results in a 4–14 D error in the IOL power in pediatric eyes, which is much higher than the 3–4 D/mm error seen in adult eyes. Besides, every diopter of error in keratometry induces a 0.8–1.3 D error in pediatric eyes.[12]

Axial length measurement is performed using ultrasonic method or optical biometry. Immersion ultrasonic technique is more accurate than applanation technique, with about 50% of eyes having an absolute prediction error of <0.5 D as compared to only 23% of the eyes using the contact method.[13]

Optical biometers are more accurate and repeatable, and it is recommended to replace the A-scan ultrasound with an optical biometer whenever feasible in view of it being a non-contact procedure with better accuracy and ease of use. Performing an optical biometry may not be possible in infants or toddlers, as it requires patient cooperation and fixation. In such cases, performing A-scan, preferably using immersion method is recommended. Keratometry for the infants and younger children is usually performed under general anesthesia using a handheld automated keratometer, though errors can be caused due to the lack of fixation and centration.[14]

INTRAOCULAR LENS POWER FORMULA

The IOL power formulae used in pediatric patients are based on theoretical or regression models developed using data from adult eyes. The AL in pediatric eyes is usually shorter, keratometry steeper, and anterior chamber depth shallower compared to adult eyes, which makes these formulae inherently less accurate.

In adult eyes, Hoffer Q, Haigis, and Holladay 2 have been reported to be more accurate for shorter ALs among the older formulae, while EVO 2.0 formula, Kane formula, Pearl-DGS, and ray tracing-based approaches have been found to be more accurate among the newer formulae.[15,16] The accuracy of these formulae cannot be extrapolated to pediatric eyes due to the difference in the optical geometry. The reported mean error in IOL power calculation in the pediatric eyes is higher and more variable ranging from 0.3 to 4.6 D as compared to 0.05–0.5 D reported in adult eyes.[17-20] The prediction error is higher and more variable in younger children and those with shorter ALs.[21]

The refractive outcomes with the theoretical third generation as well as regression formulae have been largely unsatisfactory.[17,18] In children younger than 2 years and AL <22 mm (including extremely short eyes with AL <20 mm), SRK-T, Holladay 1, and Holladay 2 perform better among the third- and fourth-generation formulae. Among the newer formulae, EVO 2.0 formula has shown better outcomes followed by Kane formula.[22,23] Interestingly, few studies report SRK-II formula to outperform the third-generation formulae.[20,24] Hoffer Q has not been found to be as accurate in this age group with a higher prediction error and a tendency for overcorrection as compared to other third-generation and regression formulae.[18,21,24]

In children above 2 years with average AL, SRK-T, Haigis, Hoffer Q, Holladay 1, and Holladay 2 performed better among the older formulae.[22,25-27] Few studies report better outcomes with SRK II formula as compared to third-generation formulae.[18,24] Among the newer formulae, Barret II universal tends to perform better in the older children with average AL along with EVO 2.0 and Kane formulae.[26,28]

POSTOPERATIVE REFRACTIVE GOAL

Postoperative refractive error after pediatric cataract surgery is determined by the targeted refractive error and prediction error, along with the AL elongation. There is no clear consensus at present regarding the ideal postoperative target in pediatric cataract surgery. Any one of the following three initial refractive goals, namely myopic, hyperopic, or emmetropic, may be aimed on a case-to-case basis. Initial myopic target provides good spectacle-free focus at near and a reduced risk of developing amblyopia, but with the tradeoff of a very high myopia when the patient reaches adulthood. Initial emmetropia may help reduce the risk of amblyopia in the immediate postoperative period but will result in moderate to high myopia in the later years requiring high minus glasses, contact lens use, or even IOL exchange. Undercorrection with resultant initial hyperopia has the advantage of a low myopia or emmetropia in adulthood, but will require stringent measures to tackle the initial hyperopia with glasses or contact lens to prevent amblyopia.[2] The most commonly used approach is to leave the child hyperopic in anticipation of the subsequent myopic shift. While deciding upon the postoperative target refraction, one should take into consideration the age at the time of surgery, laterality, refractive error of the fellow eye, and psychosocial factors such as compliance to contact lens, spectacles, and amblyopia therapy. While undergoing unilateral surgery, the surgeon may consider shifting the initial refractive goal closer to that of the fellow eye, whether emmetropic or ametropic in order to minimize aniseikonia. However, it must be emphasized to the parents that unexpected growth may occur in pseudophakic eye over the years.[29]

More hyperopia can be targeted in a bilateral surgery, as chances of amblyopia are lesser compared to unilateral pseudophakic patient who is noncompliant with glasses. Parental refractive error should also be considered, as a child with both parents myopic has about 40% chances of being myopic and may be left more hyperopic. As discussed earlier, the myopic shift seen in infants is higher and more unpredictable as compared to older children, which necessitates a higher undercorrection in this age group.

Most studies reporting the outcomes of pediatric cataract surgery with IOL implantation in infancy have used about 20–30% initial undercorrection as they have reported a myopic shift of about 5–7 D. The maximum change is observed in the first year after surgery with a substantial variance noted among the patients.[5,30] Various authors have proposed guidelines regarding the immediate postoperative refractive target for different ages, with higher values of undercorrection planned for the younger patients. **Table 1** details some of the recommended guidelines for target refraction in pediatric cataract.[5,31-34]

Enyedi et al. proposed the "Rule of 7" for IOL power undercorrection, such that the sum of postoperative hyperopic refraction and the age at surgery equals 7.[31] Acceptable visual outcomes have been reported with this method in patients <7 years, with 47.6% having final refractive error within 1 D at 7 years of age. The myopic shift was observed to be significantly lower in children <2 years of age at the time of surgery, and lower planned target hyperopia was recommended in this age group.[35]

Dahan et al. recommended a 20% undercorrection of emmetropic IOL power for children <2 years, and 10% undercorrection for children between 2 and 8 years, in order to achieve emmetropia by late childhood or a moderate myopia by adulthood.[6]

TABLE 1: Guidelines for target postoperative refractive error for children of different ages undergoing cataract surgery with intraocular lens (IOL) implantation

Age at surgery	Enyedi et al. (1998)	Plager et al. (2002)	Trivedi and Wilson (2009)	Crouch et al. (2002)	Buckley et al. (1993)	Dahan et al. (1997)-IOL power undercorrection	VanderVeen et al.* (2022)
<3 months							+10 D or no IOL
3–6 months							+8 D or no IOL
<1 years						20%	+7 D
1 year	+6 D		+6 D	+4 D	+3 D	20%	+6 D (12–18 months)
2 years	+5 D		+5 D	+3.5 D		10%	+5 D (18–24 months)
3 years	+4 D	+5 D		+2.5 D	+2 D	10%	+4 D (2–3 years)
4 years	+3 D	+4 D	+4 D	+2.5 D		10%	+3 D (3–4 years)
5 years	+2 D	+3 D	+3 D	+2 D	+1.5 D	10%	+2 D (4–5 years)
6 years	+1 D	+2.25 D	+2 D	+2 D		10%	+1 D (5–6 years)
7 years	Plano	+1.5 D	+1.5 D	+1 D	+1 D	10%	+0.5 D
8 years	−1 to −2 D	+1 D	+1 D	+1 D		10%	0.5 D
10 years	−1 to −2 D		+0.5 D	Plano	Plano	Plano	+0.25 D (8–10 years)

*Target refraction to be adjusted as follows if average K <42.5 D: +1D (2–4 years), +0.75 D (4–5 years), +0.5 D (5–8 years), +0.25 D (8–10 years).

Knight and Nanan suggested subtracting 6 D from the emmetropic IOL power in infants, 3 D for 1-4 years age group, and 1 D for 5-12 years age group.[36]

Hutchison et al. recommended implantation of emmetropic IOL power for children above 6 years of age, while subtracting 1-2 D in 3-5 years age group.[37] Chen et al. recommend deducting 1.25 D from the power needed to attain the spherical equivalent of the fellow eye for children between 2 and 4 years age, and IOL power to match the spherical equivalent of the fellow eye for those above 4 years.[38] Astle et al. recommended underpowering the IOL power by 7-8 D for children aged 1-2 years and by 5-7 D for those aged 2-4 years.[39]

The IATS used an undercorrection of 8 D for infants aged 28-48 days, and 6 D for those aged 49-210 days.[21] Based on the 5-year refractive outcomes, the authors suggested an immediate postoperative target of 10.5 and 8.5 D in the two age groups, respectively, to achieve emmetropia by 5 years of age. The authors emphasized the possibility of unexpected anisometropia in later life due to high variability in the refractive outcomes.[40] Trivedi et al. published a predictive model which uses the age of patient and AL at surgery to calculate a predicted AL at 18 years of age, which can be used to calculate the IOL power needed to achieve the desired refraction.[41]

INTRAOCULAR LENS POWER CALCULATION IN SPECIAL SCENARIOS

Secondary IOL implantation in a child is planned when the child becomes intolerant to contact lens or spectacle use or when functional vision without the use of additional correction is desired. The target hyperopia is lower in these children as they usually undergo surgery after the age of 2 years.

Factors determining the power of the IOL implanted include age at the time of IOL implantation, refractive status of the fellow eye, and the site of IOL implantation.[42] A fairly accurate assessment of the visual potential, presence of amblyopia, and strabismus is usually possible in these patients as they are older. Moreover, biometry may be more accurate if optical biometry is possible. Aphakic refraction can also be performed to estimate the IOL power, though most authors recommend the use of biometry for IOL power calculation. In the cases of unilateral pseudophakia, biometry should be performed for the fellow eye too.

The concept of temporary polypseudophakia for infants was introduced by Wilson et al. where they described the placement of two IOLs: one permanent IOL in the bag and the other temporary IOL in the sulcus. It was planned for infants who were contact-lens intolerant or unlikely to use spectacle correction for aphakia. The aim was to make the child emmetropic postsurgery (+2 to +3 D hyperopia if age <2 months) with mild myopia developing in the following 2-3 years. This prevented the child from being hyperopic during the amblyogenic age group. The power of the anterior sulcus-fixated piggyback IOL was about one-third of the total IOL power. The temporary IOL removal was planned if high myopia resulted with the increasing age or when the predicted postoperative refraction reached emmetropia on removal of the temporary IOL.[43] Boisvert et al. devised a *Pediatric Piggyback IOL Calculator* for choosing IOL power combinations for temporary polypseudophakia. They recommended an initial postoperative target of moderate hyperopia with the anterior IOL having approximately 20% of the total required IOL power for optimal outcomes. The anterior IOL may be removed once the child's myopic error equals half the anterior IOL power.[44]

The refractive prediction error in children undergoing secondary IOL implantation is higher than that seen in adults and comparable to children undergoing primary IOL implantation, with younger age groups showing higher error.[45] The IATS reported secondary IOL implantation when performed after 4.5 years of age to be more predictable than primary IOL implantation.[46]

■ CONCLUSION

Intraocular lens power calculation in children is more challenging than in adults due to a variety of factors, including the unpredictable growth of the eye after surgery, lack of IOL formula devised specifically for pediatric eyes and errors in biometry. Postoperative target refraction should be decided based on the patient's age, laterality of cataract, family history of myopia, and compliance to amblyopia treatment. Most surgeons prefer to target hyperopia in anticipation of the myopic shift after the surgery, which is higher and more variable in the younger age groups and in patients with higher-powered IOLs in situ. With the existing IOL power formulae, the prediction error remains high in these patients, especially in the younger age group. Though no formula has achieved accuracy rates comparable to adult eyes, relatively better results have been achieved with Holladay 1, Holladay 2, SRK-T, and EVO 2.0, especially in the eyes with shorter ALs. Among newer formulae, Barrett Universal II performs better in the average AL eyes and children >2 years age.

CLINICAL CASE EXAMPLES

■ CASE 1

A 10-month-old baby was referred for congenital cataract in the left eye. The right eye had a normal red reflex with a refractive error of +3 D. The biometry of both eyes was as follows:

Parameter	OD	OS
Axial length	21.5 mm	20 mm
Keratometry	47.5 D/46 D × 95°	49.0 D/47 D × 85°
Corneal diameter	11 mm	10.5 mm

The IOL power in the left eye calculated using SRK-T formula was 29.0 D. A 20% undercorrection (5.8 D) was performed and a 23 D single-piece IOL was implanted in the bag. The postoperative refraction in left eye after surgery was +5 D. The child was provided with +7 D glasses in left eye (includes +2 D near add) and was advised patching of right eye for 3–4 waking hours.

■ CASE 2

A 3-year-old child was referred for bilateral congenital cataract. The biometry of both eyes was as follows:

Parameter	OD	OS
Axial length	21.5 mm	21.4 mm
Keratometry	46 D/45 D × 90	45 D/44 D × 90
Corneal diameter	11 mm	11 mm

The IOL power in OD and OS calculated using SRK-T formula was 25.5 D and 26.5 D, respectively. Approximately 10% undercorrection of +2.5 D was performed in both eyes. The postoperative refraction in both eyes after surgery was +3 D. The child was provided with a correction of 3 D for distance and near add of 3 D (bifocal glasses) in both eyes as she was going to start playschool.

REFERENCES

1. Gordon RA, Donzis PB. Refractive development of the human eye. Arch Ophthalmol. 1985;103:785-9.
2. McClatchey SK, Hofmeister EM. The optics of aphakic and pseudophakic eyes in childhood. Surv Ophthalmol. 2010;55:174-82.
3. Trivedi RH, Wilson ME, Bandyopadhyay D. Refractive shift in pseudophakic eyes during the second decade of life. J Cataract Refract Surg. 2012;38:102-7.
4. Lambert SR, Nizam A, DuBois L, Cotsonis G, Weakley DR Jr, Wilson ME; Infant Aphakia Treatment Study Group. The myopic shift in aphakic eyes in the infant aphakia treatment study after 10 years of follow-up. Eye Contact Lens. 2021;47:108-12.
5. VanderVeen DK, Oke I, Nihalani BR. Deviations from age-adjusted normative biometry measures in children undergoing cataract surgery: Implications for postoperative target refraction and IOL power selection. Am J Ophthalmol. 2022;239:190-201.
6. Dahan E, Drusedau MU. Choice of lens and dioptric power in pediatric pseudophakia. J Cataract Refract Surg. 1997;23(Suppl 1):618-23.
7. Hoevenaars NED, Polling JR, Wolfs RCW. Prediction error and myopic shift after intraocular lens implantation in paediatric cataract patients. Br J Ophthalmol. 2011;95:1082-5.
8. Zhou X, Fan F, Liu X, Yang J, Yang T, Luo Y. The impact of pre-operative axial length on myopic shift 3 years after congenital and developmental cataract surgery and intraocular lens implantation. Front Med (Lausanne). 2022;9:1093276.
9. Wilson ME, Trivedi RH, Weakley DR, Cotsonis GA, Lambert SR; Infant Aphakia Treatment Study Group. Globe axial length growth at age 5 years in the Infant Aphakia Treatment Study. Ophthalmology. 2017;124:730-3.
10. Plager DA, Lynn MJ, Buckley EG, Wilson ME, Lambert SR; Infant Aphakia Treatment Study Group. Complications in the first 5 years following cataract surgery in infants with and without intraocular lens implantation in the Infant Aphakia Treatment Study. Am J Ophthalmol. 2014;158:892-8.
11. Mittelviefhaus H, Gentner C. [Errors in keratometry for intraocular lens implantation in infants]. Ophthalmologe. 2000;97:186-8.
12. Eibschitz-Tsimhoni M, Tsimhoni O, Archer SM, Del Monte MA. Effect of axial length and keratometry measurement error on intraocular lens implant power prediction formulas in pediatric patients. J AAPOS. 2008;12:173-6.
13. Trivedi RH, Wilson ME. Prediction error after pediatric cataract surgery with intraocular lens implantation: Contact versus immersion A-scan biometry. J Cataract Refract Surg. 2011;37:501-5.
14. Trivedi RH, Wilson ME. Keratometry in pediatric eyes with cataract. Arch Ophthalmol. 2008;126:38-42.
15. Hoffer KJ, Savini G. IOL power calculation in short and long eyes. Asia Pac J Ophthalmol (Philadelphia). 2017;6:330-1.
16. Vilaltella M, Cid-Bertomeu P, Huerva V. Accuracy of 10 IOL power calculation formulas in 100 short eyes (≤22 mm). Int Ophthalmol. 2023;43:2613-22.
17. Mezer E, Rootman DS, Abdolell M, Levin AV. Early postoperative refractive outcomes of pediatric intraocular lens implantation. J Cataract Refract Surg. 2004;30:603-10.
18. Neely DE, Plager DA, Borger SM, Golub RL. Accuracy of intraocular lens calculations in infants and children undergoing cataract surgery. J AAPOS. 2005;9:160-5.
19. Nihalani BR, VanderVeen DK. Comparison of intraocular lens power calculation formulae in pediatric eyes. Ophthalmology. 2010;117:1493-9.
20. Kekunnaya R, Gupta A, Sachdeva V, Rao HL, Vaddavalli PK, Om Prakash V. Accuracy of intraocular lens power calculation formulae in children less than two years. Am J Ophthalmol. 2012;154:13-19.e2.

21. Vanderveen DK, Trivedi RH, Nizam A, Lynn MJ, Lambert SR; Infant Aphakia Treatment Study Group. Predictability of intraocular lens power calculation formulae in infantile eyes with unilateral congenital cataract: results from the Infant Aphakia Treatment Study. Am J Ophthalmol. 2013; 156:1252-60.e2.
22. Chang P, Lin L, Li Z, Wang L, Huang J, Zhao YE. Accuracy of 8 intraocular lens power calculation formulas in pediatric cataract patients. Graefes Arch Clin Exp Ophthalmol. 2020;258(5):1123-31.
23. Yılmaz İE, Kimyon S, Mete A. Challenges in pediatric cataract surgery: comparison of intraocular lens power calculation formulas using optical biometry. Int Ophthalmol. 2022;42:3071-7.
24. Lee BJ, Lee S-M, Kim JH, Yu YS. Predictability of formulae for intraocular lens power calculation according to the age of implantation in paediatric cataract. Br J Ophthalmol. 2019;103:106-11.
25. Zhong Y, Yu Y, Li J, Lu B, Li S, Zhu Y. Accuracy of intraocular lens power calculation formulas in pediatric cataract patients: a systematic review and meta-analysis. Front Med (Lausanne). 2021;8:710492.
26. Lin L, Fang J, Sun W, Gu S, Xu L, Chen S, et al. Accuracy of newer generation intraocular lens power calculation formulas in pediatric cataract patients. Graefes Arch Clin Exp Ophthalmol. 2023;261:1019-27.
27. Kou J, Chang P, Lin L, Li Z, Fu Y, Zhao YE. Comparison of the accuracy of IOL power calculation formulas for pediatric eyes in children of different Ages. J Ophthalmol. 2020;2020:8709375.
28. Hong Y, Sun Y, Xiao B, Ainiwaer M, Ji Y. A Bayesian network meta-analysis on comparisons of intraocular lens power calculation methods for paediatric cataract eyes. Eye (London). 2023;37:3313-21.
29. McAllum P, Rootman D. Paediatric intraocular lenses: the power to choose? Clin Experiment Ophthalmol. 2007;35:201-2.
30. Lambert SR, Buckley EG, Plager DA, Medow NB, Wilson ME. Unilateral intraocular lens implantation during the first six months of life. J AAPOS. 1999;3:344-9.
31. Enyedi LB, Peterseim MW, Freedman SF, Buckley EG. Refractive changes after pediatric intraocular lens implantation. Am J Ophthalmol. 1998;126:772-81.
32. Crouch ER, Crouch ER Jr, Pressman SH. Prospective analysis of pediatric pseudophakia: myopic shift and postoperative outcomes. J AAPOS. 2002;6:277-82.
33. Buckley EG, Klombers LA, Seaber JH, Scalise-Gordy A, Minzter R. Management of the posterior capsule during pediatric intraocular lens implantation. Am J Ophthalmol. 1993;115:722-8.
34. Plager DA, Kipfer H, Sprunger DT, Sondhi N, Neely DE. Refractive change in pediatric pseudophakia: 6-year follow-up. J Cataract Refract Surg. 2002;28:810-5.
35. Sachdeva V, Katukuri S, Kekunnaya R, Fernandes M, Ali MH. Validation of guidelines for undercorrection of intraocular lens power in children. Am J Ophthalmol. 2017;174:17-22.
36. Flitcroft DI, Knight-Nanan D, Bowell R, Lanigan B, O'Keefe M. Intraocular lenses in children: changes in axial length, corneal curvature, and refraction. Br J Ophthalmol. 1999;83:265-9.
37. Hutchinson AK, Drews-Botsch C, Lambert SR. Myopic shift after intraocular lens implantation during childhood. Ophthalmology. 1997;104:1752-7.
38. Eibschitz-Tsimhoni M, Archer SM, Del Monte MA. Intraocular lens power calculation in children. Surv Ophthalmol. 2007;52:474-82.
39. Astle WF, Ingram AD, Isaza GM, Echeverri P. Paediatric pseudophakia: analysis of intraocular lens power and myopic shift. Clin Exp Ophthalmol. 2007;35:244-51.
40. Weakley DR, Lynn MJ, Dubois L, Cotsonis G, Wilson ME, Buckley EG, et al. Myopic shift 5 years after intraocular lens implantation in the Infant Aphakia Treatment Study. Ophthalmology. 2017;124:822-7.
41. Trivedi RH, Barnwell E, Wolf B, Wilson ME. A model to predict postoperative axial length in children undergoing bilateral cataract

surgery with primary intraocular lens implantation. Am J Ophthalmol. 2019;206: 228-34.
42. Sachdeva V, Reddy P, Fernandes M, Shah S, Kekunnaya R. Refractive outcomes with secondary intraocular lens implantation in children. J AAPOS. 2010;14:377-8.
43. Wilson ME, Peterseim MW, Englert JA, Lall-Trail JK, Elliott LA. Pseudophakia and polypseudophakia in the first year of life. J AAPOS. 2001;5(4):238-45.
44. Boisvert C, Beverly DT, McClatchey SK. Theoretical strategy for choosing piggyback intraocular lens powers in young children. J AAPOS. 2009;13:555-7.
45. Moore DB, Ben Zion I, Neely DE, Roberts GJ, Sprunger DT, Plager DA. Refractive outcomes with secondary intraocular lens implantation in children. J AAPOS. 2009;13: 551-4.
46. VanderVeen DK, Drews-Botsch CD, Nizam A, Bothun ED, Wilson LB, Wilson ME, et al. Outcomes of secondary intraocular lens implantation in the Infant Aphakia Treatment Study. J Cataract Refract Surg. 2021;47:172-7.

CHAPTER 12

Intraocular Lens Power Calculation in Corneal Pathologies

INTRODUCTION

Cataract surgery may be required in patients with various corneal pathologies, including corneal ectasia, corneal scars, dystrophies, and prior keratoplasty. Precise intraocular lens (IOL) power calculation in irregular corneas is extremely challenging, and the refractive outcomes remain unpredictable.

The corneal pathology may be progressive in nature as in ectasia and endothelial dystrophies. In addition, present-day instruments may not accurately assess the corneal power in irregular corneas and extremes of corneal curvature. The choice of IOL is complicated by the presence of irregular astigmatism. We discuss the challenges faced in IOL power calculation and various methods to achieve accurate biometry and precise IOL power in these cases.

INTRAOCULAR LENS POWER CALCULATION IN CORNEAL ECTASIA

Corneal ectatic disorders are characterized by bilateral, noninflammatory thinning and steepening of the cornea, leading to irregular astigmatism and progressive vision loss.[1] Vernal keratoconjunctivitis and chronic eye rubbing are frequently associated with keratoconus. The propensity to develop cataract is higher than normal in cases with corneal ectasia, owing to prolonged use of topical corticosteroids, associated atopy, ocular comorbidities, and ocular surgeries in addition to the age-related senile cataract.[2,3]

Challenges in Accurate Biometry and IOL Power Calculation in Corneal Ectasia

Intraocular lens power calculation in keratoconus patients is challenging and associated with unpredictable results **(Table 1)**. Difficulties are faced during axial length estimation, keratometry, and prediction of the effective lens position (ELP). In addition, an irregular tear film further compounds errors during biometry. Conventional IOL power calculation formulae have low predictability in ectatic corneas.

Axial Length

Keratoconus is often associated with axial elongation and myopia. The corneal apex in ectasia is decentered, and an accurate estimation of the visual axis may be uncertain and challenging. Alió et al. observed that the post-cataract surgery residual spherical equivalent in keratoconus had a stronger correlation with axial length than with keratometry, thereby highlighting the significance of accurate axial length estimation.[4]

TABLE 1: Challenges in IOL power calculation in keratoconus

Parameters	Challenges	Preferred modality
Axial length	• Longer than usual • Decentered corneal apex—does not coincide with visual axis	Optical biometers
Keratometry	• Overestimation of keratometry • Altered anterior to posterior corneal curvature ratio, irregular cornea with asymmetric astigmatism, irregular tear film, deep ACD	• Mild–moderate keratoconus—optical biometers, Scheimpflug tomographers • Keratometry centered over pupil rather than corneal vertex—more accurate • Severe keratoconus—use standard K (43.5 D)
IOL power formulae	• Underestimate IOL power • Postoperative hyperopic surprise • Prediction of ELP inaccurate	• SRK/T—most accurate • Barret Universal II, Kane KC, SRK II (mild disease), Haigis (severe disease) • Target postoperative myopia—more with advanced disease • Low predictability of all formulae in advanced disease

(ACD: anterior chamber depth; ELP: effective lens position; IOL: intraocular lens)

Keratometry

Keratometry is overestimated in cases with corneal ectasia, leading to postoperative hyperopia. Conventional placido disk-based corneal topography devices employ certain assumptions to calculate the corneal curvature and power, including a fixed relation between the anterior and posterior corneal curvature. The assumptions do not hold true in ectatic corneas and lead to inaccurate estimation of keratometry.[5-7] The following errors are encountered during measurement of corneal curvature:

- *Index of refraction error:* The ratio of anterior to posterior corneal curvature is altered in ectasia, and the normal keratometric index of 1.3375 to derive corneal power is inaccurate.
- *Instrument error:* The conventional Placido disk-based keratometers are unable to measure corneal power accurately, owing to asymmetric corneal curvature and steep corneas. The corneal power varies along a given meridian and is not constant. In addition, the two principal meridians are not perpendicular to each other. The visual axis and corneal apex often do not coincide.
- *Irregular tear film:* The tear-film distribution over a thinned steep cornea is also irregular, owing to decreased accuracy and repeatability of keratometry measurements.

IOL Power Calculation Formulae

All IOL power calculation formulae underestimate the IOL power to variable extents and result in postoperative residual hyperopia. Newer regression formulae incorporate ELP to enhance accuracy, which in turn is determined by anterior chamber depth (ACD), white to white, and axial length. The usual relationship between corneal curvature, ACD, and IOL position is disrupted in keratoconus, thus reducing the accuracy of ELP estimation by the IOL power calculation formula.

Intraocular lens power calculation for toric IOLs is specially challenging, as there may be poor repeatability in both the magnitude and axis of toricity with increasing disease severity.[8,9]

Prior to performing cataract surgery, it is of utmost importance to confirm disease stability and establish the stage of disease in these patients. The three important components of IOL power calculation in keratoconus patients include accurate axial length measurement, corneal power assessment, and use of appropriate IOL power calculation formula.

Prerequisites Before Intraocular Lens Power Calculation in Ectasia

It is essential to ascertain cataract as the cause for vision loss and document disease stability before proceeding with cataract surgery in a case with keratoconus.

Ascertain the Cause of Vision Loss

Both keratoconus and cataract are characterized by progressive loss of vision, and it is essential to determine that the cataract is visually significant before proceeding with surgery. Rigid gas-permeable lenses with over-refraction may compensate for the vision loss due to keratoconus in mild–moderate disease, and the proportion of vision loss due to cataract can be reliably assessed. In advanced disease with significant central corneal scarring, the surgeon may consider performing keratoplasty before proceeding with cataract surgery.

Document Stability

It is essential to document stability of keratoconus by comparing topographical maps and indices obtained at least 6–12 months apart. Cataract surgery in progressive keratoconus will lead to suboptimal results and a dissatisfied patient. In cases of unstable disease, collagen cross linking should be performed if the corneal thickness is within the specified range.

Counseling

Patient counseling is of paramount importance in patients with keratoconus undergoing cataract surgery. Patient expectations should be addressed, and a realistic overview of the expected refractive outcomes should be provided. The need for postoperative spectacles and contact lenses to obtain optimal visual acuity and quality should also be explained to the patient. The type of IOL planned for implantation should also be discussed, and the patients should be counseled against multifocal IOLs.

Timing of Biometry

Majority of patients with corneal ectasia may already be using contact lenses, and a lens-free interval is essential to negate the effect of contact lens-induced corneal warpage and obtain accurate biometry. For soft contact lenses, at least 1 week off contact lenses is recommended. For rigid gas-permeable lenses, hybrid or toric lenses, the interval ranges from 2 to 3 weeks. For scleral lenses not touching the cornea, 2–3 days is adequate before obtaining biometry measurements.

Biometry and IOL Power Calculation

Optical biometers and elevation-based topography devices provide more reliable axial length and keratometry measurements. Various IOL power calculation formulae have been evaluated, and the outcomes vary with the disease severity **(Flowchart 1)**.

Axial Length

Ultrasonic biometry is inaccurate in keratoconus as the visual axis and corneal

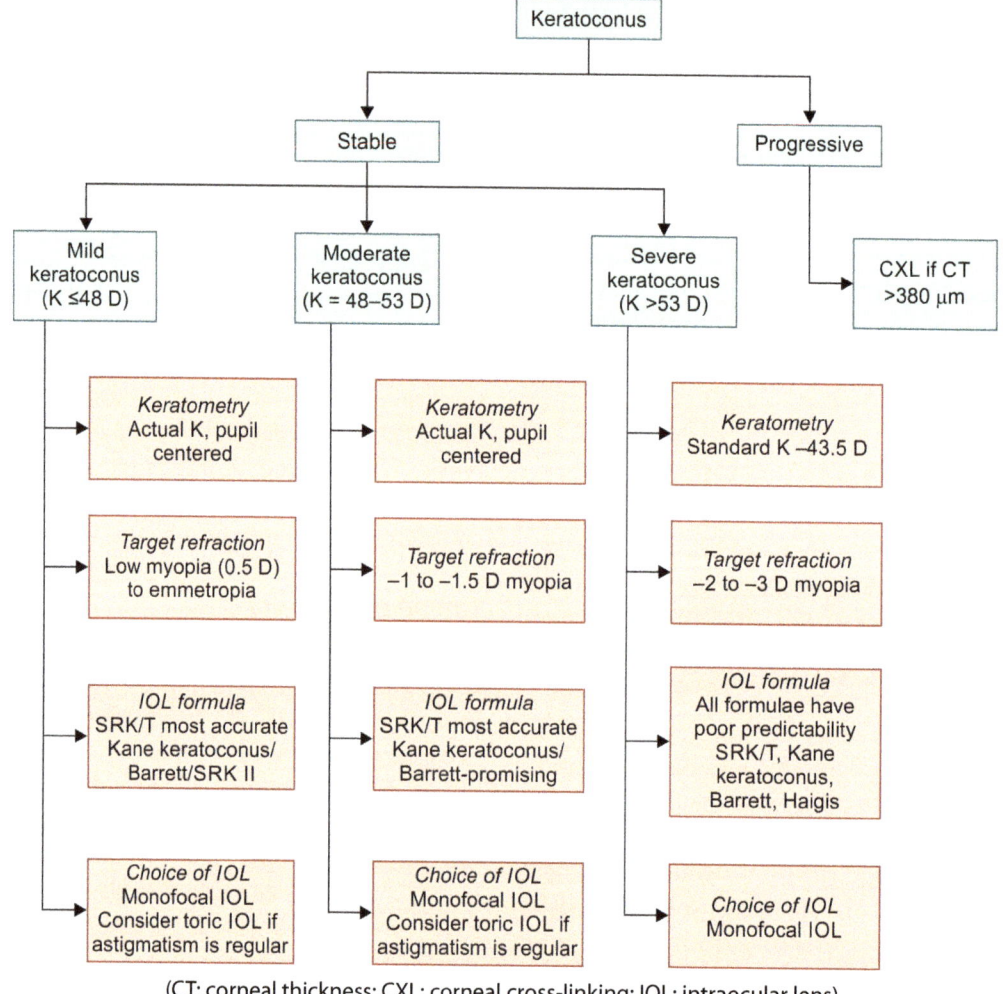

Flowchart 1: Management algorithm for IOL power calculation in keratoconus

(CT: corneal thickness; CXL: corneal cross-linking; IOL: intraocular lens)

apex may not coincide.[4,10] Optical biometry is preferred for axial length measurement as the estimation of visual axis is more accurate.

Keratometry

Manual and automated keratometers have low reliability in keratometry estimation and should be avoided. Keratometry readings from Placido disc topographer have been observed to be steeper than the Pentacam sim K values in keratoconus.[11]

Both the anterior and posterior corneal curvature should be considered while estimating the corneal power. Swept-source optical coherence tomography (OCT) based optical biometers provide accurate keratometry readings in mild–moderate disorders. True K values (accounting for posterior corneal curvature) should be preferred over keratometry obtained from the anterior corneal surface alone.

Elevation-based topography devices, such as Scheimpflug-camera-based devices

(Pentacam, Galilei) provide an accurate estimate of the true corneal power.[12] Various maps are available in these devices, including true net power (TNP), total corneal refractive power (TCRP), and equivalent K readings (EKR), which take into account both the anterior and posterior corneal curvature.[13] Of note, TNP and TCRP are calculated using a refractive index of 1.376 and may not be directly used with conventional IOL power calculation formulae such as SRK/T (Sanders–Retzlaff–Kraff theoretical), Hoffer Q, and Holladay 1; however, EKR values may be directly used with these formulae **(Fig. 1)**. The zone in which the corneal power is calculated may also be determined and customized, and pupil-centered measurements may be preferred over vertex-centered measurements in cases with significantly decentered corneal apex **(Fig. 2)**.[13]

In mild-to-moderate keratoconus, the actual keratometry readings obtained with any of the newer devices are fairly accurate, and Watson et al. observed 60% of eyes with mild keratoconus (<48 D) and 41.9% eyes with moderate keratoconus (>48 and <55 D) to be within 1 D of target postoperative refractive error.[14]

In cases with advanced keratoconus, with K >55 D, none of the available devices has acceptable accuracy, and taking a standard K of 43.5 D for IOL power calculation has been advised.[14,15]

IOL Power Calculation

All IOL power calculation formulae are associated with post-cataract surgery hyperopic refractive outcomes in keratoconus. The third-generation theoretical formulae estimate the ELP based on AL (axial length)

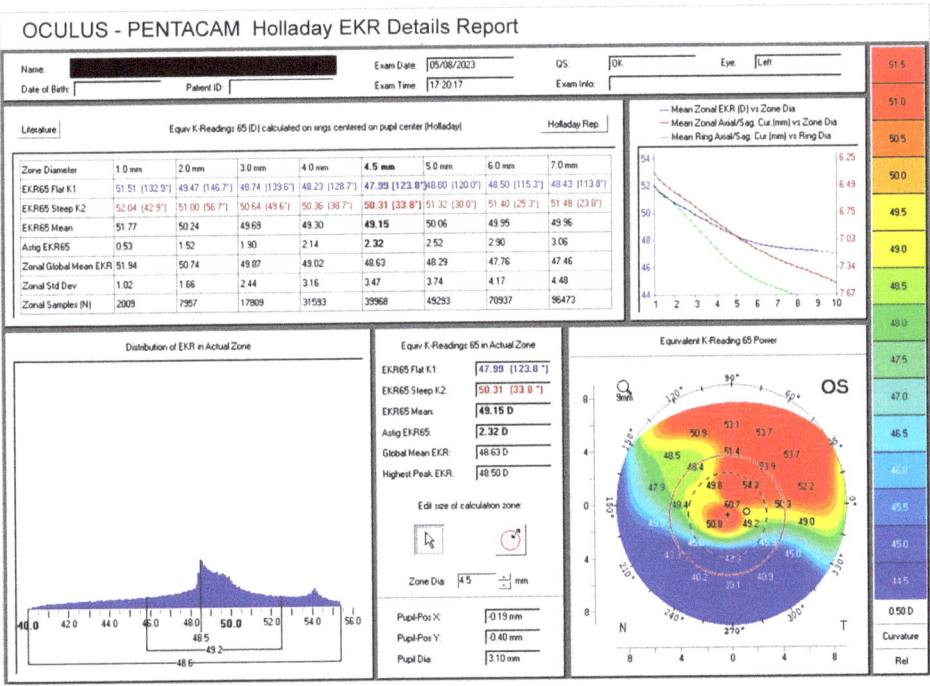

Fig. 1: Equivalent K readings (EKR) obtained using Scheimpflug topography (Pentacam) take into account both the anterior and posterior corneal curvature. EKR values may be directly used with regression formulae such as SRK/T, Hoffer Q, and Holladay 1

OCULUS - PENTACAM Corneal Power Distribution

K-Readings (D) calculated on rings centered on vertex

Ring Diameter	1.0 mm	2.0 mm	3.0 mm	4.0 mm	5.0 mm	6.0 mm	7.0 mm	8.0 mm
Axial / Sagittal Front Km	54.5	53.2	51.7	50.2	49.3	48.5	47.4	45.5
Astig	6.4 (99.6°)	4.3 (98.3°)	1.9 (93.2°)	0.5 (67.7°)	0.4 (69.6°)	0.8 (118.1°)	1.7 (145.3°)	3.2 (158.6°)
True Net Power Km	52.0	50.9	49.5	48.3	47.7	47.2	46.3	44.5
Astig	6.3 (99.5°)	4.0 (99.0°)	1.6 (94.7°)	0.6 (64.2°)	0.8 (71.0°)	1.1 (96.3°)	1.1 (130.1°)	2.3 (157.4°)
Tot. Refr. Power Km	52.9	52.0	50.9	50.2	50.2	50.6	50.7	49.7
Astig	6.2 (99.2°)	4.0 (98.3°)	1.6 (92.5°)	0.6 (58.0°)	1.0 (70.6°)	1.7 (95.1°)	1.8 (123.6°)	3.2 (155.3°)

K-Readings (D) calculated on rings centered on pupil center

Ring Diameter	1.0 mm	2.0 mm	3.0 mm	4.0 mm	5.0 mm	6.0 mm	7.0 mm	8.0 mm
Axial / Sagittal Front Km	51.7	49.9	49.0	48.0	47.2	46.7	46.4	45.9
Astig	0.8 (110.5°)	1.8 (105.4°)	1.9 (102.6°)	0.9 (103.6°)	0.4 (123.0°)	1.1 (119.7°)	2.6 (114.8°)	4.2 (116.6°)
True Net Power Km	49.5	47.8	47.1	46.3	45.5	45.2	45.0	44.8
Astig	0.6 (111.6°)	1.6 (104.3°)	1.7 (106.5°)	0.7 (117.8°)	0.5 (140.5°)	0.9 (115.7°)	2.5 (108.0°)	4.0 (110.9°)
Tot. Refr. Power Km	49.8	48.8	48.4	47.9	47.6	48.0	48.9	
Astig	0.2 (161.3°)	2.0 (102.3°)	1.7 (103.9°)	0.5 (119.3°)	0.5 (168.0°)	0.5 (125.0°)	2.6 (107.6°)	(110.9°)

Fig. 2: Keratometry readings centered on corneal vertex and pupil center, in a case with keratoconus. Vertex-centered measurements overestimate the keratometry values in cases with decentered corneal apex

and K, while the fourth- and fifth-generation formulae employ additional variables. Any inaccuracy in K assessment will presumably translate into an error in ELP estimation. The predictability of the third- and fourth-generation formulae, while being acceptable in cases of mild keratoconus, is rather poor in the moderate and severe cases.

Thebpatiphat et al. reported SRK II to be the most accurate formula in mild keratoconus cases among the second- and third-generation formulae.[2]

Studies evaluating the accuracy and predictability of third- and fourth-generation theoretical formulae in keratoconus eyes observed SRK/T to be the most accurate, with 36–43.9% of eyes within 0.5 D prediction error.[5,16,17] This may be explained by the tendency for postoperative myopic prediction error with SRK/T formula in steep corneas without keratoconus, which may balance the postoperative hyperopia observed in keratoconus eyes.[5,6]

Savini et al. compared the predictability of five IOL power calculation formulae in different stages of keratoconus: SRK-T, Barrett Universal II, Holladay 1, Haigis, and Hoffer Q. The stages of keratoconus were derived from the Amsler Krumeich grading, and stage I (K ≤ 48 D), stage II (K = 48–53 D), and stage III (K > 53 D) cases were included. They observed highest predictability with SRK/T formula, with 61.9% eyes with stage I, 30.77% eyes with stage II, and 14.29% eyes with stage III keratoconus within a postoperative target prediction error of 0.5 D. Both Holladay 1 and Barrett formulae were comparable, but inferior to SRK/T; Hoffer Q had the least predictability.[5]

Barrett universal II formula has been found to be fairly accurate in the stage I and II keratoconus eyes.[18] Wang et al. observed the lowest prediction error with Barrett Universal II formula in mild–moderate keratoconus and with Haigis formula in severe keratoconus.[18] Recently, modifications have been proposed in the Holladay 2 formula and Kane formula to allow their use in keratoconus eyes with greater accuracy. The Holladay IOL consultant software allows the user to designate an eye as keratoconus, thus changing the underlying ELP algorithm to account for the independence between anterior segment size and axial length. Kane keratoconus formula, a theoretical modification of the original formula, uses corneal power derived from the anterior corneal radii of curvature that better represents the true anterior/posterior ratio in keratoconus eyes and aims to minimize the effect of corneal power on the ELP calculation.

A recent study by Kane et al. reported the Kane keratoconus formula to be most accurate, with 50% of the eyes within 0.5 D of target error. Notably, it performed fairly well even in stage 3 keratoconus cases (>53 D) with a smaller mean hyperopic bias of 0.2 D, as compared to a much higher hyperopic error, ranging from 1.72 D to 3.02 D observed with other formulae.[17]

Various nomograms have been suggested regarding the choice of IOL power and target postoperative myopia based on the disease severity. It is advisable to target greater postoperative residual myopia with increasing severity of keratoconus, to compensate for the hyperopic refractive surprise.

Choice of IOL

A monofocal IOL is preferred in keratoconus eyes to achieve optimal visual quality in an aberrated cornea (Case Example 1). Toric IOLs may be implanted in case of mild or mild–moderate keratoconus, with stable disease, and a good repeatability of both the magnitude and the axis of toricity; however, the patient must be appropriately counseled beforehand that the purpose of the toric IOLs is to reduce the burden of cylinder power and not completely eliminate it (Case Example 2).[4,8,9]

Multifocal IOLs, extended depth of focus IOLs, and monofocal IOLs with enhanced intermediate vision should be avoided in cases with keratoconus, as the dysphotopsia, reduced contrast, and aberrations induced by these IOLs may lead to a significant deterioration of the visual quality in these eyes.

INTRAOCULAR LENS POWER CALCULATION AND KERATOPLASTY

Cataract surgery may need to be performed prior to, simultaneously, or sequentially after a keratoplasty procedure. IOL power calculation is challenging in each of these aforementioned scenarios. In addition, the type of procedure, whether full thickness, anterior lamellar or endothelial keratoplasty (EK), also impacts the IOL power calculation.

Challenges in Biometry and IOL Power Calculation

Cataract surgery in keratoplasty may be performed simultaneously with the keratoplasty ("triple" procedure) or as a sequential procedure. In eyes undergoing simultaneous triple procedure, accurate prediction of postoperative corneal power may not be feasible and remains a major source of error. Corneal transplantation changes the constants assumed by the conventional theoretical formulae, notably the ratio of the anterior–posterior corneal curvature to ACD.

In patients undergoing EK, posterior corneal curvature is predominantly modified by the surgery and significantly influences the corneal power and the IOL power calculated. The endothelial graft in Descemet stripping automated endothelial keratoplasty (DSAEK) has a meniscus-shaped configuration and is thicker in the periphery, which leads to steepening of the posterior surface with increased posterior corneal curvature.[19] The ratio of posterior to anterior corneal radius of curvature is reduced in post-DSAEK eyes compared to normal eyes.

Keratometry Estimation and IOL Power Calculation

Post-phacoemulsification visual and refractive outcomes after full-thickness keratoplasty are relatively guarded, especially in combined procedures. Accurate IOL power calculation in EK is less challenging, and majority of new-generation IOL power formulae with modern-day topographers and tomographers provide precise outcomes.

Full-thickness or Anterior Lamellar Keratoplasty

In eyes undergoing simultaneous penetrating keratoplasty (PK) or lamellar keratoplasty (LK) with cataract surgery, standard keratometry value of 43.5 D, contralateral keratometry, or a mean K value derived from the surgeon's past keratoplasties may be used to calculate the IOL power with any of the new-generation IOL power calculation formulae. There is a tendency for postoperative hyperopia with resultant poor uncorrected visual acuity after full-thickness triple procedures.[20] In contrast, visual outcomes after combined DALK with phacoemulsification are relatively better, with 62.8% having corrected distance visual acuity of 0.3 logMAR or better.[21] Accuracy of IOL power calculation is better when cataract surgery is performed in a sequential manner rather than as a simultaneous procedure.

In patients undergoing sequential cataract surgery after PK or LK, complete suture removal and stabilization of refractive error prior to cataract surgery are preferred.[22] Optical biometry for axial length assessment and computerized topography for estimation of central corneal power should be performed whenever possible. Pellegrini et al. observed a tendency for myopic shift after cataract surgery in post-DALK cases, with increased predictability with Kane, EVO, Hoffer QST, and SRK/T formulae.[23]

Endothelial Keratoplasty

Ray-tracing methods and Scheimpflug-based devices that measure both anterior and posterior corneal curvature provide an accurate estimate of true corneal power after EK.[24] Xu et al. observed accurate results using EKR at 4 mm for IOL power calculation after DSAEK.[25] Diener et al. proposed an adjustment of the conventional keratometric index based on the ratio of postoperative posterior corneal curvature to preoperative anterior corneal curvature in eyes planned for DMEK triple.[26]

Posterior corneal steepening and regression of corneal edema after EK result in a hyperopic shift of about +1.5 D. In patients undergoing DSAEK triple or cataract surgery prior to EK, this hyperopic shift must be taken into account during IOL power calculation by targeting for a myopic outcome. A similar but lower hyperopic shift of about 0.32 D is seen after Descemet membrane endothelial keratoplasty (DMEK). Knutsson et al. observed comparable refractive outcomes with newer generation IOL power calculation formulae after DMEK, including Barrett Universal II, EVO 2.0, Haigis, Hoffer Q, Holladay 1, Kane, and SRK/T formulae.[27] Optimization of the ULIB constants further improves accuracy.[27]

Choice of IOL

Aspheric monofocal IOLs are preferred in patients with keratoplasty. Post-keratoplasty high astigmatism of >5 D magnitude may be observed in 15–31% of patients, and toric IOLs are the procedure of choice in cases with regular orthogonal astigmatism.[28,29] Prerequisites for implanting a toric IOL include prior complete suture removal, stable refractive error over the past 6 months to 1 year, and regular astigmatism.

High irregular astigmatism may be observed in up to two-third cases after PK.[30] Monofocal IOLs should be preferred in irregular astigmatism, and postoperative use of rigid gas-permeable contact lens helps to achieve optimal visual outcomes.

INTRAOCULAR LENS POWER CALCULATION IN CORNEAL SCARS

Various methods have been described to assess corneal power in patients with corneal scar. Contact lens over-refraction using a hard contact lens has been described for corneal power assessment in corneal scar cases with a visual acuity of 20/70 or better; this is especially useful in irregular astigmatism.

Conventional keratometers may give fallaciously high K readings in cases with central corneal scars, as the flattening in the scarred region is surrounded by a paracentral region of steepening. Irregular mires are observed with severe corneal scarring, and reliable keratometry readings may not be obtained.

Newer corneal topography and tomography devices based on Scheimpflug imaging and LED technology are more accurate for anterior corneal surface assessment in highly irregular corneas.[31] Alteration of the anterior to posterior corneal curvature ratio is observed in cases with predominantly anterior corneal scarring; devices that directly measure both anterior and posterior corneal surfaces are more accurate in such cases (Case Example 3).

CONCLUSION

To conclude, IOL power calculation in corneal pathologies is challenging, with a tendency toward overestimation of keratometry and underestimation of IOL power, resulting in postoperative hyperopic surprise. Accurate biometry measurements may be achieved with newer optical biometry devices and elevation-based topographers taking into account both the anterior and posterior corneal curvature.

Accurate postoperative outcomes are observed with new-generation IOL power calculation formulae. SRK-T has been found to be most predictable IOL power calculation formula in mild–moderate keratoconus, with fairly reliable outcomes also observed with Barrett II, Holladay, and Kane KC formulae. In cases with severe keratoconus, no device or formula is accurate. A standard K of 43.5 D may be used for calculations and target myopia of 2–3 D to minimize postoperative hyperopia.

Monofocal IOLs are preferred and toric IOLs may be implanted in select cases with stable mild disease and relatively regular corneas. Patient counseling is a must to ensure postoperative satisfaction, and the need for postoperative spectacles or contact lenses should be emphasized.

CLINICAL CASE EXAMPLES

CASE 1

A 35-year-old-female patient with advanced keratoconus with intumescent cataract in both eyes was planned for cataract surgery in the right eye. The keratometry was stable since the past 2 years.

Pre-cataract surgery parameters (right eye):

AL	25.48 mm
ACD	3.85 mm
LT	4.11 mm
WTW	12.2 mm
K1/K2 (sim K from Pentacam)	54.3 D @ 30°/57.6 D @ 120°

(ACD: anterior chamber depth; AL: axial length; LT: lens thickness: WTW: white-to-white)

- IOL power calculated (targeting –1.3 D myopia) with Barrett Universal II formula = –1 D
- IOL power calculated (targeting –1.3 D myopia) with SRK-T formula = –5 D
- Patient was implanted with –1 D monofocal IOL
- Postoperative uncorrected distant visual acuity (UCDVA) was 6/24 P with a refraction of +2.5 DS –4 DC@103°

■ CASE 2

A 19-year-old-male patient with bilateral keratoconus and posterior subcapsular cataract was planned for cataract surgery in the right eye. The keratometry was stable since past 2 years.

Pre-cataract surgery parameters (right eye):

AL	23.23 mm
ACD	4.14 mm
LT	2.7 mm
WTW	12.8 mm
K1/K2 (sim K from Pentacam)	42.27 D @ 5°/47.6 D @ 95°

- Patient was planned for toric monofocal IOL implantation (targeting –0.34 D myopia)
- IOL power calculated using Barrett Universal II formula.
- Patient was implanted with 21.5 D (T9) Alcon AcrySof IQ Toric IOL aligned at 96° axis.
- Postoperative UCDVA was 6/9 and best spectacle-corrected visual acuity (BSCVA) was 6/6 with acceptance of +0.75 DC × 95°.

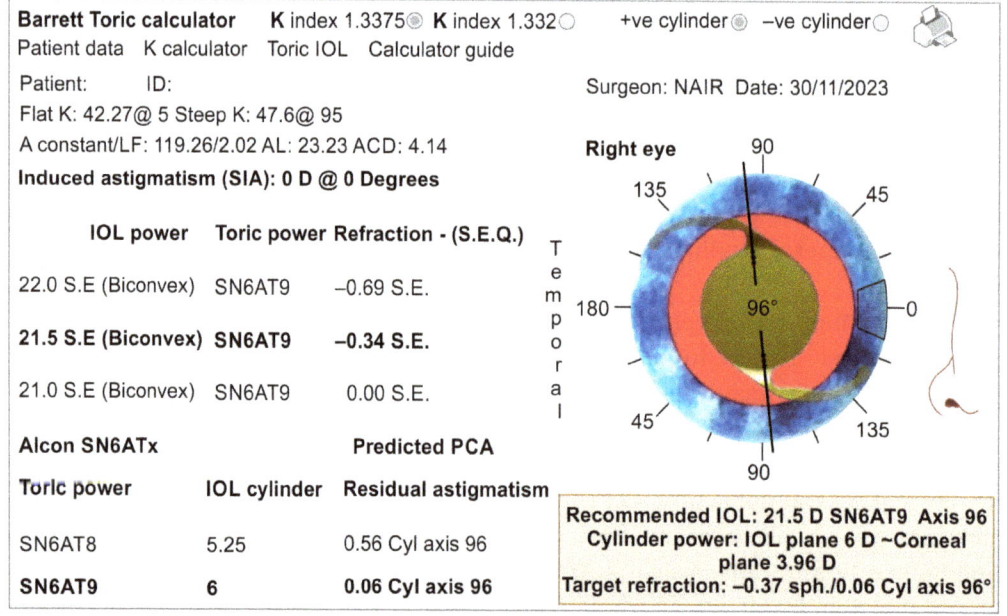

CHAPTER 12: Intraocular Lens Power Calculation in Corneal Pathologies

CASE 3

A 65-year-old-male patient with a peripheral leucomatous corneal opacity and cataract was planned for phacoemulsification with posterior chamber IOL implantation in the right eye.

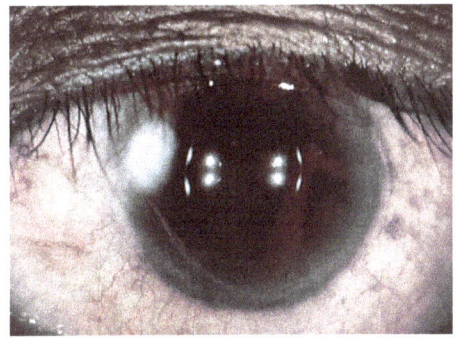

Pre-cataract surgery parameters (right eye):

AL	23.65 mm
ACD	3.22 mm
LT	4.12 mm
K1/K2 (Placido-disk topography)	41.65 D @ 95°/42.88 D @ 172°
K1/K2 (IOLMaster 700)	41.46 D @ 75°/42.93 D @ 165°

In view of peripheral location of corneal opacity with repeatable keratometry readings on different devices, the patient was planned for a toric IOL implantation and IOL power calculation was performed using Barrett Toric Calculator.

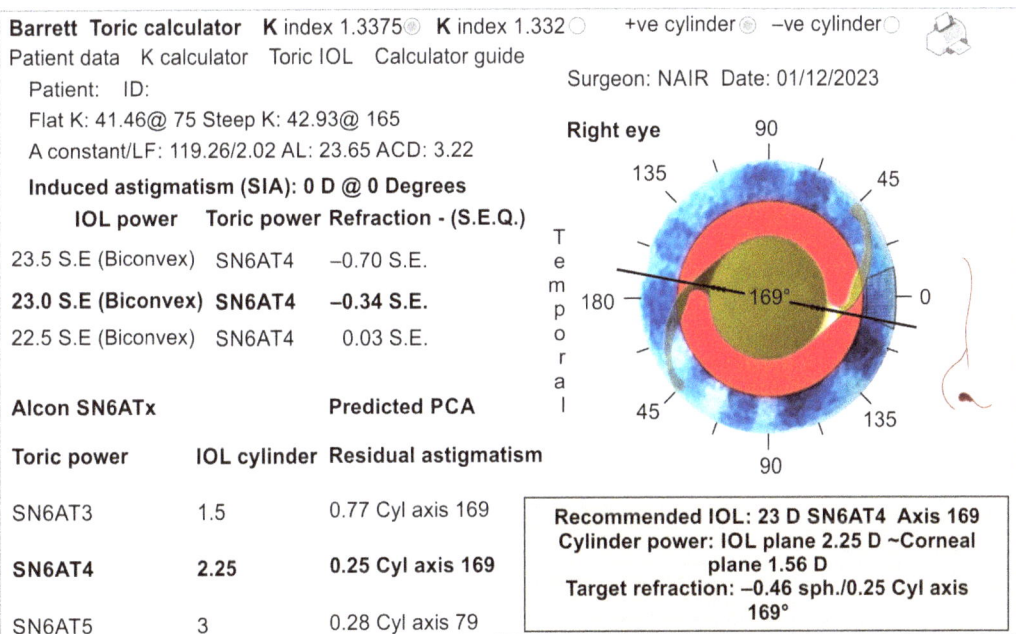

- Patient was implanted with 23 D (T4) Alcon AcrySof IQ Toric IOL aligned at 169° axis.
- Postoperative UCDVA was 6/9 and BSCVA was 6/6 with acceptance of −0.5 DC × 95°.

REFERENCES

1. Santodomingo-Rubido J, Carracedo G, Suzaki A, Villa-Collar C, Vincent SJ, Wolffsohn JS. Keratoconus: An updated review. Cont Lens Ant Eye. 2022;45:101559.

2. Thebpatiphat N, Hammersmith KM, Rapuano CJ, Ayres BD, Cohen EJ. Cataract surgery in keratoconus. Eye Contact Lens. 2007;33:244-6.
3. Leccisotti A. Refractive lens exchange in keratoconus. J Cataract Refract Surg. 2006;32:742-6.
4. Alió JL, Peña-García P, Abdulla Guliyeva F, Soria FA, Zein G, Abu-Mustafa SK. MICS with toric intraocular lenses in keratoconus: outcomes and predictability analysis of postoperative refraction. Br J Ophthalmol. 2014;98:365-70.
5. Savini G, Abbate R, Hoffer KJ, Mularoni A, Imburgia A, Avoni L, et al. Intraocular lens power calculation in eyes with keratoconus. J Cataract Refract Surg. 2019;45:576-81.
6. Ghiasian L, Abolfathzadeh N, Manafi N, Hadavandkhani A. Intraocular lens power calculation in keratoconus; A review of literature. J Curr Ophthalmol. 2019;31:127-34.
7. Singh C, Joshi VP. Cataract surgery in keratoconus revisited - An update on preoperative and intraoperative considerations and postoperative outcomes. Semin Ophthalmol. 2023;38:57-64.
8. Jaimes M, Xacur-García F, Alvarez-Melloni D, Graue-Hernández EO, Ramirez-Luquín T, Navas A. Refractive lens exchange with toric intraocular lenses in keratoconus. J Refract Surg. 2011;27:658-64.
9. Hashemi H, Heidarian S, Seyedian MA, Yekta A, Khabazkhoob M. Evaluation of the Results of Using Toric IOL in the Cataract Surgery of Keratoconus Patients. Eye Contact Lens. 2015;41:354-8.
10. Yağcı R, Güler E, Kulak AE, Erdoğan BD, Balcı M, Hepşen IF. Repeatability and reproducibility of a new optical biometer in normal and keratoconic eyes. J Cataract Refract Surg. 2015;41:171-7.
11. Saglik A, Celik H, Aksoy M. An Analysis of Scheimpflug Holladay-Equivalent Keratometry Readings Following Corneal Collagen Cross-Linking. Beyoglu Eye J. 2019;4:62-8.
12. Chalkiadaki E, Gartaganis PS, Ntravalias T, Giannakis I, Manousakis E, Karmiris E. Agreement in anterior segment measurements between swept-source and Scheimpflug-based optical biometries in keratoconic eyes: a pilot study. Ther Adv Ophthalmol. 2022;14:25158414211063283.
13. Kim J, Whang W-J, Kim H-S. Analysis of total corneal astigmatism with a rotating Scheimpflug camera in keratoconus. BMC Ophthalmol. 2020;20:475.
14. Watson MP, Anand S, Bhogal M, Gore D, Moriyama A, Pullum K, et al. Cataract surgery outcome in eyes with keratoconus. Br J Ophthalmol. 2014;98:361-4.
15. Hashemi H, Yekta A, Khabazkhoob M. Effect of keratoconus grades on repeatability of keratometry readings: Comparison of 5 devices. J Cataract Refract Surg. 2015;41:1065-72.
16. Kamiya K, Iijima K, Nobuyuki S, Mori Y, Miyata K, Yamaguchi T, et al. Predictability of Intraocular Lens Power Calculation for Cataract with Keratoconus: A Multicenter Study. Sci Rep. 2018;8:1312.
17. Kane JX, Connell B, Yip H, McAlister JC, Beckingsale P, Snibson GR, et al. Accuracy of Intraocular Lens Power Formulas Modified for Patients with Keratoconus. Ophthalmology. 2020;127:1037-42.
18. Wang KM, Jun AS, Ladas JG, Siddiqui AA, Woreta F, Srikumaran D. Accuracy of Intraocular Lens Formulas in Eyes With Keratoconus. Am J Ophthalmol. 2020;212:26-33.
19. Clemmensen K, Ivarsen A, Hjortdal J. Changes in Corneal Power After Descemet Stripping Automated Endothelial Keratoplasty. J Refract Surg. 2015;31:807-12.
20. Claoué C, Ficker L, Kirkness C, Steele A. Refractive results after corneal triple procedures (PK+ECCE+IOL). Eye Lond Engl. 1993;7(Pt 3):446-51.
21. Alfonso-Bartolozzi B, Fernández-Vega-Cueto L, Fernández-Vega L, Martínez-Alberquilla I, Madrid-Costa D, Alfonso JF. Triple Procedure: A Stepwise Combination of Deep Anterior Lamellar Keratoplasty and Cataract Surgery. Cornea. 2023. doi: 10.1097/ICO.0000000000003364.

22. Dietrich T, Viestenz A, Langenbucher A, Naumann GOH, Seitz B. [Accuracy of IOL power prediction in cataract surgery after penetrating keratoplasty–retrospective study of 72 eyes]. Klin Monatsbl Augenheilkd. 2011;228:698-703.
23. Pellegrini M, Furiosi L, Salgari N, D'Angelo S, Zauli G, Yu AC, et al. Accuracy of intraocular lens power calculation for cataract surgery after deep anterior lamellar keratoplasty. Clin Experiment Ophthalmol. 2022;50:17-22.
24. Alnawaiseh M, Zumhagen L, Rosentreter A, Eter N. Intraocular lens power calculation using standard formulas and ray tracing after DMEK in patients with Fuchs endothelial dystrophy. BMC Ophthalmol. 2017;17:152.
25. Xu K, Qi H, Peng R, Xiao G, Hong J, Hao Y, et al. Keratometric measurements and IOL calculations in pseudophakic post-DSAEK patients. BMC Ophthalmol. 2018;18:268.
26. Diener R, Treder M, Lauermann JL, Eter N, Alnawaiseh M. Assessing the validity of corneal power estimation using conventional keratometry for intraocular lens power calculation in eyes with Fuch's dystrophy undergoing Descemet membrane endothelial keratoplasty. Graefes Arch Clin Exp Ophthalmol Albrecht Von Graefes Arch Klin Exp Ophthalmol. 2021;259:1061-70.
27. Knutsson KA, Savini G, Hoffer KJ, Lupardi E, Bertuzzi F, Taroni L, et al. IOL Power Calculation in Eyes Undergoing Combined Descemet Membrane Endothelial Keratoplasty and Cataract Surgery. J Refract Surg. 2022;38:435-42.
28. Feizi S, Zare M. Current Approaches for Management of Postpenetrating Keratoplasty Astigmatism. J Ophthalmol. 2011;2011: 708736.
29. Lockington D, Wang EF, Patel DV, Moore SP, McGhee CNJ. Effectiveness of cataract phacoemulsification with toric intraocular lenses in addressing astigmatism after keratoplasty. J Cataract Refract Surg 2014; 40:2044-9.
30. Karabatsas C, Cook S, Sparrow J. Proposed classification for topographic patterns seen after penetrating keratoplasty. Br J Ophthalmol. 1999;83:403-9.
31. Kanellopoulos AJ, Asimellis G. Clinical Correlation between Placido, Scheimpflug and LED Color Reflection Topographies in Imaging of a Scarred Cornea. Case Rep Ophthalmol. 2014;5:311-7.

CHAPTER 13

Intraocular Lens Power Calculation in Posterior Segment Pathology

■ INTRODUCTION

Patients with posterior segment pathologies often develop cataract as a part of their disease process as well as surgical interventions. Intraocular lens (IOL) power calculation in these cases is challenging, owing to various factors. Firstly, anatomical factors such as macular edema, epiretinal membrane (ERM), or rhegmatogenous retinal detachment (RRD) result in errors in axial length (AL) assessment. Biometry may also be influenced by the presence of a scleral buckle, encircling band, or silicone oil (SO)/gas tamponade. Poor visual acuity and visual potential of these eyes impair accuracy of biometry and assessment of postoperative refractive outcomes.

In this chapter, we discuss the challenges and sources of error in performing accurate biometry in cases with posterior segment pathologies, and methods to improve predictability of IOL power calculation.

■ INTRAOCULAR LENS POWER CALCULATION AND SCLERAL BUCKLING

Nearly 38% eyes undergoing scleral buckling develop cataract within the first year of surgery.[1] Biometric parameters including AL, anterior chamber depth (ACD), and corneal astigmatism undergo a continual change after scleral buckling, with maximal impact on AL **(Table 1)**.

- The shape of the globe changes from spherical to prolate, resulting in elongation of AL in the majority of cases. Less frequently, high indent and scleral invagination at the buckle site may result in shortening of the AL. A 0.57–0.98 mm increase in AL is observed, with the maximal increase in the initial 3–6 months. The rate of AL elongation decreases or stabilizes in the late postoperative period and may even decrease slightly though still remaining higher than the baseline.[2-5]

TABLE 1: Changes in biometry after scleral buckling

Biometric parameter	Change
Shape of globe	Change from spherical to prolate
Axial length	0.57–0.98 mm increase (maximal in initial 3–6 months)
Anterior chamber depth	0.08–0.5 mm decrease (maximum in initial 6–9 months)
Corneal curvature	0.43–1.5 D increase (maximum in initial 3 months, stabilizes by 6–12 months)
Refractive status	−1.04 to −2.93 D myopic shift (stabilizes by 3 months)

Higher AL elongation has been observed with circumferential buckles, extensive segmental buckling, and cryotherapy as compared with encirclage band alone.[3,5,6] No difference has been observed between a silicone sponge and solid silicone element.[6]

- Reduction in ACD after scleral buckling is attributed to the vitreous compression induced by the buckle with forward displacement of lens-iris diaphragm.[7] The ACD reduction ranges from 0.08 to 0.5 mm with maximum reduction in the early postoperative period of 6-9 months, followed by stabilization or variable increase in the late postoperative period.[2,3,7,8]
- Corneal curvature increase of 0.43-1.5 D is observed in the initial 3 months, followed by a decrease, with a trend toward returning to preoperative values by 6-12 months postsurgery.[2,9] Local segmental buckles induce astigmatism, with the astigmatic axis corresponding to that of the buckle.[10] Encircling elements usually result in a more regular astigmatism with a coupled steep and flat axis.
- Most studies report a significant myopic shift after scleral buckling, ranging from −1.04 to −2.93 D, which stabilizes by 3 months postoperatively.[2,6,7] Postoperative myopic refractive shift is attributed majorly to the increase in AL, with contribution by other factors such as anterior displacement of lens-iris diaphragm, increased lens thickness due to ciliary body contraction, and corneal curvature changes.[5,7]

Intraocular lens power calculation is significantly affected by the combined effect of change in AL and ACD. Most third-generation formulae calculate the ELP based on AL and Km, which may not be accurate after scleral buckling. It is imperative to wait for the biometric parameters to stabilize before planning a cataract surgery after scleral buckling. The refractive error and ACD stabilize first followed by AL. Stabilization of AL is expected by 3-9 months post-buckling, with a recent long-term analysis reporting a slower increase in AL after the initial 6 months (0.02 mm/month after 6 months compared with 0.15 mm/month in the first 6 months).[2-4]

Simultaneous cataract surgery with scleral buckling may be performed; however, IOL power calculation should account for postoperative induced myopia which may range from 1 to 2 D with encircling band or buckle. Evaluation of post-buckling AL by the surgeon may help derive a personalized "surgeon factor" to estimate the myopic shift.[11]

INTRAOCULAR LENS POWER CALCULATION IN SILICONE-OIL-FILLED EYES

Cataract is observed in nearly 100% of eyes after SO injection with SO retained for 6 months or more.[12] Cataract surgery may be planned with the SO remaining in situ, as a combined procedure with silicone oil removal (SOR).

IOL Power Calculation in Eyes Planned for Silicone Oil Removal

Staged or simultaneous cataract surgery may be performed in patients planned for SOR, based on the grade of cataract, intraoperative posterior segment visualization, and need for further posterior segment intervention. Studies have observed variable results with the two approaches, with Krepler et al. reporting similar outcomes with combined or sequential approaches and Madanagopalan et al. observing more accurate refractive outcomes with SOR followed by phacoemulsification.[13,14]

Refractive outcomes of simultaneous cataract surgery in oil-filled eyes undergoing SOR are variable, with some studies revealing a hyperopic error[15,16] while others showing a myopic error.[17] Suk et al. observed mean myopic predictive error with both A-scan and partial coherence interferometry (PCI) and suggested targeting hyperopia of 0.5–1.25 D in patients undergoing combined phaco-SOR.[17]

Axial length assessment is the most challenging aspect in accurate IOL power calculation in oil-filled eyes, with various calculations and methods described to enhance predictive accuracy.

Methods for Axial Length Estimation (Table 2)

- Ultrasonic AL is fallaciously high in the presence of SO in situ, as the velocity of sound in SO is slower (987 m/sec in 1,000 centistokes SO) than that in vitreous (1,532 m/sec).[15] *Changing the sound speed in vitreous cavity (VC) to 987 m/sec in the biometry machine helps in accurate measurement of AL*, with predictable results reported in eyes without high myopia planned for combined phaco-SOR.[16] The attenuation of sound beam in oil-filled eyes may lead to weak retinal echo, with the strong scleral echo being mistaken for the retinal echo. This may be avoided by keeping the beam as perpendicular as possible to the ocular surface with a sufficiently high gain.[18]
- Hoffer[19] suggested measuring the AL in phakic eyes filled with SO at a speed of 1,000 m/s. The true AL is then calculated using an equation wherein 1,139 m/sec

TABLE 2: Axial length measurement in oil-filled eyes

Measurement method	Description
Ultrasonic methods	Change sound speed in vitreous cavity to 987 m/sec in ultrasound machine
	Hoffer et al. measure AL at 1,000 m/sec AL_{true} = AL at 1,000 × 1,139/1,000
Conversion factors	$AL_{corrected}$ = AL measured at 1,532 m/sec × 0.71
	$AL_{corrected}$ = Length of AC + LT + 0.64 × VC length
	Add the lengths of AC, LT, and VC, each calculated separately based on different velocities of sound in each of them
	AL (mm) = Length of (AC + Lens) + (VC × 0.634) + RSS
Intraoperative measurement	*Intraoperative measurement* of AL after SOR using ultrasonic methods
	Intraoperative aphakic refraction IOL Power = R × 2.01449
	Actual power of IOL using AIR = IOL power predicted using A-scan × 0.94 – 2.6
Fellow eye axial length	Limited utility in anisometropia or one-eyed patients
Pre-vitrectomy AL	Limited use in cases with macula-off RD/surgical intervention like encirclage/buckle
Optical biometers (IOLMaster/Lenstar)	10 × increased accuracy

(AC: anterior chamber; AIR: automated intraoperative refraction; AL: axial length; LT: lens thickness; R: spherical equivalent calculated corrected for a vertex distance of 50 cm; RSS: retrosilicone space; VC: vitreous cavity) is considered as the velocity of sound through a phakic eye filled with SO:

$$AL_{true} = AL \text{ at } 1{,}000 \times 1{,}139/1{,}000$$

- Various *conversion factors* may be applied to conventional AL measurements obtained using standard speed.[15]

$$AL_{corrected} = AL_{measured\ at\ 1{,}532\ m/s} \times 0.71$$

  - The conversion factor of 0.71 was described for 1,300 centistokes SO, and accuracy may be adversely affected by the type of oil used, under filled eyes, coloboma/staphyloma, and cases with macula-off retinal detachment (RD).
  - Larkin et al. described a conversion factor of 0.64 for the VC length. The corrected VC length is then added to the A-scan-derived length of anterior chamber (AC) and lens thickness (LT):[12]

$$AL_{corrected} = \text{Length of AC} + LT + 0.64 \times VC \text{ length}$$

  - Meldrum's formula calculates AL by adding the lengths of AC, LT, and VC, each calculated separately based on the different velocities of sound in each of them.[20]
  - An oil-free space has been observed behind the SO and in front of the macular area, termed the retro-silicone space (RSS), which is largest in the supine position and least in the prone position.[21] Nepp et al. take into account the RSS measured using immersion A-scan:

$$AL\ (mm) = \text{Length of (AC + Lens)} + (\text{vitreous length} \times 0.634) + RSS$$

  The speed of sound waves in RSS is assumed to be the same as that in vitreous. Nepp et al. observed the mean length of RSS to be 1.9 mm, and neglecting it resulted in a deviation from the target error by >5 D.[18]

- *Intraoperative measurement* of AL may be performed after SOR in eyes undergoing combined phaco-SOR. Accuracy may be affected by poor patient fixation due to the effect of the peribulbar block or adverse anatomical features such as fundal coloboma or posterior staphyloma.
  - *Intraoperative aphakic refraction* after SO removal can aid in IOL power calculation, bypassing the need to measure the AL or keratometry. Patwardhan et al.[22] performed intraoperative manual retinoscopy after SOR and cataract extraction, using the formula suggested by Ianchulev et al. to calculate the IOL power:[23]

$$\text{IOL power} = R \times 2.01449$$

  where R is the standard error (SE) calculated corrected for a vertex distance of 50 cm.
  - A regression formula based on automated intraoperative refraction (AIR) has been described for IOL power calculation after SOR and cataract extraction:

  Actual power of IOL using AIR = IOL power predicted using A-scan × 0.94 – 2.6

  The mean postoperative refraction undergoes a myopic shift from 0.53 D at 1 week to 0.12 D at 3 months. The initial hyperopic error is attributed to the lower IOP in the myopic vitrectomized eyes in the immediate postoperative period.
- *Fellow eye AL* may be used for IOL power calculation. A mean difference of 0.4 mm has been reported between the SO-filled eye and the contralateral eye; 46% of eyes had an inter-eye difference of <0.3 mm while 26% had >1 mm difference.[18]

- The method is of limited utility in anisometropia or one-eyed patients.
- Using the *previtrectomy AL* has been suggested; it is of limited use in cases with macula off RD and surgical interventions such as use of an encirclage/buckle or vitrectomy, which in itself causes AL elongation.[16]
- *Optical biometers* such as IOLMaster and Lenstar have enhanced the accuracy of AL measurement in oil-filled eyes by up to 10 times. IOLMaster uses a mean refractive index, which takes into account the presence of SO while measuring the AL, with reliable measurements obtained even in eyes with posterior staphyloma or longer ALs.[24]

IOL Power Calculation in Eyes Not Planned for Silicone Oil Removal

Cataract surgery in oil-filled eyes using conventional formulae is associated with a postoperative hyperopia of +4 to +5.4 D, owing to a higher refractive index of SO (1.405) compared to the vitreous (1.336). The refractive power of the posterior surface of a biconvex IOL is determined by the difference in the refractive index of the IOL material [1.47 for polymethyl methacrylate (PMMA); 1.41–1.55 for hydrophobic acrylic] and that of the substance in the VC. This difference is smaller when SO occupies the VC instead of vitreous, resulting in a reduced optical power and a more hyperopic residual error.[25] The curvature of the front surface of SO is determined by the SO volume and may also affect the final refractive outcomes.

Choice of IOL: Convexo-concavo or a meniscus-shaped IOL is the ideal shape to minimize the postoperative hyperopic shift; a plano-convex IOL also results in a smaller hyperopic error than a biconvex lens.[26] IOL with a lower refractive index and a steeper posterior convex side results in a higher hyperopic error when SO is injected into pseudophakic eyes. Silicone IOL material should be avoided as SO may interact with IOL material causing opacification. Plano-convex PMMA or acrylic IOLs have less interaction with SO and are preferred.

IOL power and target error: If the SO is intended to be left in situ permanently, the expected hyperopic shift should be accounted for while calculating the IOL power. Liu et al. suggested targeting –3 D myopia to partially compensate for the SO-induced hyperopia.[27] The hyperopic residual error may also be accounted for by adding a correction quotient [67.4/(AL – 4.6) D] to the calculated IOL power.[18,20]

INTRAOCULAR LENS POWER IN COMBINED PHACOVITRECTOMY PROCEDURES

Cataract formation is observed in up to 80% of the eyes undergoing pars plana vitrectomy (PPV) within the first 2 years after surgery.[1] Combined phacovitrectomy helps in faster visual rehabilitation, better surgical visualization, and cost effectiveness. IOL power calculation remains a challenge, with studies showing variable degrees of residual refractive error, mostly myopic, after combined cataract surgery and PPV.

Challenges in IOL Power Calculation

Intraocular lens power calculation is performed using standard formulae, and there are currently no dedicated IOL power formulae customized for patients undergoing vitrectomy. A myopic shift is observed after combined phacovitrectomy, with erroneous AL measurement being the most important causative factor. Other contributory factors include change in ELP or ACD, effect of gas tamponade, formula-induced error, surgeon factor, IOL type, change in keratometry, types of macular pathology, surgical technique, and preoperative myopic RE.

- *Inaccurate AL measurement* is the most significant causative factor for IOL power calculation errors, with 100 μm underestimation of AL resulting in 0.25–0.28 D myopic shift.[28] Myopic predictive error has been observed with the use of both acoustic biometry and optical-based biometry, including the newer swept-source optical coherence tomography (SS-OCT)-based devices.[29,30] Ultrasonic AL estimation is less accurate than optical methods, owing to the corneal compression induced during indentation which is more pronounced in high myopic eyes. Changes in macular thickness result in erroneous measurements, and the increased echogenicity of a thick ERM, foveal detachment, or detached perifoveal cuff may all result in false low readings.[31] Inadequate fixation due to poor vision can lead to erroneous measurements by both optical and ultrasonic methods but may affect the PCI-based measurements more as they depend on proper fixation for accuracy.[31]
- Myopic shift may also be related to a *true increase in the postoperative AL*. Cho et al. hypothesized the postoperative increase in AL to be related to the normalization of IOP in eyes undergoing PPV for RRD, which are usually hypotonous before surgery.[32] Jee et al. observed a larger myopic shift in high myopic eyes (>26 mm) post vitrectomy, which they attributed to a true increase in AL and keratometry documented 4 months postoperatively using an optical biometer. Thinner sclera and lower ocular rigidity in high myopia increase the susceptibility of these eyes to globe deformation post surgery.[33]
- A significant deepening of AC has been observed after combined phacovitrectomy, and the increase may be greater than observed after routine phacoemulsification.[34] A higher postoperative predictive error has been observed in patients with shallow preoperative ACD, as there is a greater potential for change in ACD due to zonular stretch in these cases, thereby increasing the variability in ELP.[29]
- The *effect of gas tamponade on the ELP* and hence the refractive outcome remain unclear. Most authors implicate gas tamponade in postoperative myopic shift by pushing the IOL anteriorly, thus changing the ELP due to its buoyant effect.[35] In contrast, Falkner et al. concluded that the eventual absorption of gas increased the zonular elasticity with resultant posterior shift of IOL and lesser myopic shift.[34]
- *IOL design or the type of IOL* also influences the amount of anterior shift under the influence of gas tamponade, with greater shift reported with a single piece foldable IOL as compared to a three-piece IOL. Single-piece IOLs are less resistant to subsequent capsule contraction than three-piece IOLs; angulation and 4 haptic design single-piece IOLs provided better stability.[36]
- *Retinal pathologies* like ERM[34] and macular hole (MH)[37] are a predictive factor for higher myopic shift.
- *Replacement of the vitreous with aqueous* after vitrectomy leads to a reduction in the refractive index of the VC by about 0.003, which also results in −0.13 to −0.5 D of myopic shift.[28]

Methods to Improve Refractive Outcomes

Numerous methods have been proposed to improve the accuracy of refractive outcomes in patients undergoing combined PPV and phacoemulsification.

- *Aiming for a slight hyperopic target refraction*[35] or implanting an IOL one step lower (0.5 D less) than the emmetropic power helps counter the expected myopic shift.[34]
- *Adjusted or corrected AL* may be calculated by adding the predicted change in central macular thickness (CMT) postsurgery to the preoperative ultrasonic AL. It is difficult to predict the change in CMT, and the difference between measured macular thickness and that of a normal eye or the fellow eye can be used for AL adjustment. However, persistent myopic error has been reported despite AL adjustment using these methods.[38,39]
- Using the *true refractive vitreal index* of refraction in the IOL power formulae and taking into consideration the replacement of vitreous with aqueous post-PPV may also improve the predictive accuracy.
- Newer generation IOL power calculation formulae may be more accurate. Vounotrypidis et al. compared eight IOL power calculation formulae (both third- and fourth generation) in eyes undergoing combined phacovitrectomy for ERM using a SS-OCT-based biometer and observed the highest accuracy with the Kane formula, followed by Holladay 2 and Barrett formulae.[40] *Optimization of IOL constants* helps eliminate any systematic myopic or hyperopic prediction error (PE) and is recommended while using the newer IOL calculation formulae.
- *SS-OCT-based biometry devices* enable more precise AL measurement. The use of IOL Master 700 in eyes undergoing combined phacovitrectomy results in accurate refractive outcomes comparable to routine phacoemulsification, with 70–82% of the eyes having a PE < 0.5 D and a minimal myopic shift.[30,41]
- Measuring the actual ELP immediately following cataract extraction using microscope integrated or mounted intraoperative OCT may help improve the accuracy of IOL power calculations.[42]
- Surgical techniques such as posterior capsulotomy during phacovitrectomy may help counter the tendency for postoperative myopic shift.[43]

INTRAOCULAR LENS POWER CALCULATION IN PHACOVITRECTOMY FOR RETINAL DETACHMENT

Combined phacoemulsification with PPV is often required in eyes with RRD to obtain an unimpeded view of retinal periphery. The postoperative myopic shift is greater in RRD eyes than after phacovitrectomy for other VR pathologies such as ERM or MH.[32]

Challenges in IOL Power Calculation

Error in accurate estimation of AL is the most important cause of postoperative refractive error in these eyes.

Both ultrasonic and optical biometry methods are inaccurate with underestimation of AL due to the shortening of the distance between the corneal vertex and the vitreoretinal interface of the detached retina. PCI-based optical biometers are often less successful than ultrasonic methods in acquiring an acceptable scan. A-scan ultrasonography underestimates AL in macula-off RD by up to 0.82 mm, whereas optical biometers underestimate the AL by up to 0.98 mm despite an acceptable signal to noise ratio (SNR).[44,45]

While performing applanation A-scan, the increased corneal indentation due to the hypotony often present in RRD eyes further accentuates AL errors.[32] Immersion A-scan is more accurate than PCI-based optical biometers in assessing AL in eyes with macula detached, as the supine position during ultrasonic measurement allows the SRF to disperse and decrease the height of detachment.[46] In cases with macula-on RD, both immersion A-scan and IOLMaster 500 are comparable.[46] The ability of the PCI-based biometers to capture AL in macula-off RRDs is often compromised, owing to poor fixation and interference of the detached retina with light reflectivity, resulting in signals from the detached retina rather than retinal pigment epithelium (RPE). The magnitude of error is increased with more bullous RD.

Myopic shift is seen in RRD eyes post-phacovitrectomy even when the macula is spared.[47] Other factors such as the use of gas tamponade, preoperative AC depth, and lens thickness also induce myopic shift in these eyes.

Methods to Improve Refractive Outcomes

Combination of PCI device and ultrasonic biometry (preferably immersion) may help enhance the accuracy of AL estimation (**Flowchart 1**). *User-adjusted optical biometry*

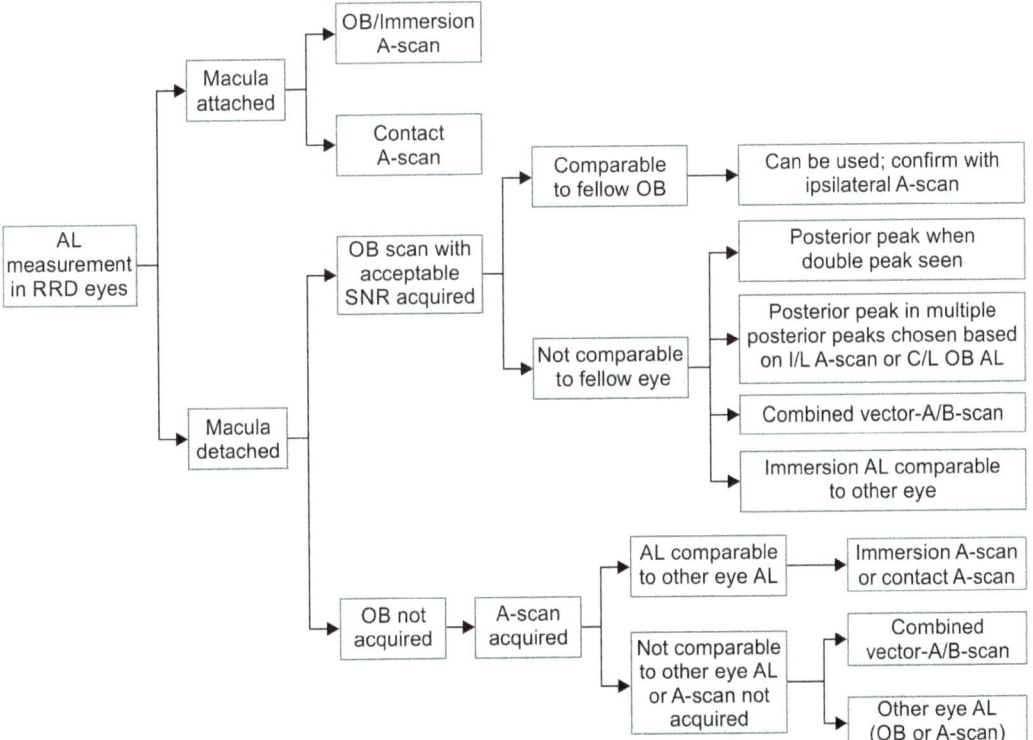

Flowchart 1: Algorithm for assessing AL in an eye with RRD

(AL: axial length; C/L: contralateral; I/L: ipsilateral; OB: optical biometry; RD: retinal detachment)

may be employed when using PCI-based optical biometers in macula-off RD, where the operator can manually select the posterior peak in cases with double peak to obtain accurate AL measurement. In cases with multiple posterior peaks, the peak giving AL values corresponding to the AL measured with A-scan or contralateral eye AL measured using PCI device may be selected. Preoperative user adjusted optical biometry (UAOB) derived AL has been observed to be comparable to preoperative A-scan measured AL and postoperative PCI biometers measured AL with retina attached. IOL power calculation accuracy in terms of percentage of eyes within 0.5 D is better with preoperative UAOB-derived AL than the A-scan AL (92% vs. 77%).[48]

Axial length measurements in eyes with macula-off should be correlated with that of the fellow eye and known refraction, whenever possible. Fellow eye AL may be used when both PCI device and A-scan measurement is shorter than the fellow eye, provided there was no significant difference in the refractive error of both eyes before RD.

Axial length measured using a *combined vector-A/B-scan (contact)* method gives more accurate AL measurements as compared to IOLMaster or contact A-scan in cases with detached macula. A two-dimensional B-scan image guides the overlying vector-A-scan to directly measure to the fovea. Immersion-combined vector-A/B-scan method may further improve the accuracy.[44]

Intraocular lens power may be adjusted to aim for postoperative hyperopia of approximately +0.5 D to counteract the myopic shift. Refractive error of the fellow eye may be taken into consideration in order to balance the postoperative residual error and prevent aniseikonia.

INTRAOCULAR LENS POWER IN POST-VITRECTOMIZED EYES

Refractive outcomes after cataract surgery in eyes that have undergone previous vitrectomy are less accurate than eyes without any previous surgery.[49] Contrary to the myopic shift observed after combined phacovitrectomy, eyes undergoing sequential cataract surgery in a vitrectomized eye usually show a hyperopic shift. This may be attributed primarily to the changes in the ACD and ELP.[49]

Wang et al. observed hyperopic shift only in vitrectomized eyes which had a gas tamponade at the time of vitrectomy. The possible mechanism was the deepening of AC with posterior shift of the IOL–bag complex due to the increased elasticity of the zonules in eyes which had previous gas tamponade.[50] Optical biometry may be more accurate in eyes with associated high axial myopia or posterior staphyloma.

Improved accuracy of the newer IOL power calculation formulae has been demonstrated in post-PPV eyes undergoing cataract surgery, with a recent study reporting Holladay 2 formula with the most accurate result. It must be emphasized that all formulae gave a hyperopic predictive error with a higher variability in outcomes than non-vitrectomized eyes.

CONCLUSION

Axial length estimation poses the major challenge in accurate IOL power calculation in eyes with various vitreoretinal pathologies. It is imperative to allow stabilization of biometric parameters after buckling/encirclage for at least 6–9 months. SO-filled eyes have a significant proportion of eyes with a residual myopic or hyperopic error, whether using ultrasound biometry or optical biometry. The use of the newer SS-OCT-based biometers may prove beneficial in these eyes, especially when associated with RD, ERM, or macular edema. Intraoperative aberrometry may be another promising option which could be used to determine the IOL power on-table after SOR and cataract extraction. New-generation IOL power formulae give fairly accurate outcomes, with sequential surgeries associated with better refractive outcomes as compared to combined procedures.

CLINICAL CASE EXAMPLES

CASE 1

A 55-year-old patient who had previously undergone vitreoretinal surgery with SO injection in his right eye was planned for cataract surgery with SOR. The ocular parameters measurement using A-scan with preset sound speed of 1,532 m/sec were as follows. The AL was not captured on optical biometry due to low SNR and dense cataract.

Pre-cataract surgery parameters (right eye):

Axial length	34.71 mm
Anterior chamber depth	2.24 mm
Lens thickness	4.37 mm
Vitreous cavity length	28 mm

The AL in the fellow eye was 22.3 mm. The corrected AL in right eye was calculated as per the formula:

$$AL_{corrected} = \text{Length of AC} + LT + 0.64 \times VC \text{ length}$$

$$AL_{corrected} = 2.24 + 4.47 + (0.64 \times 28) = 24.53 \text{ mm}$$

Intraocular lens power was calculated using Barrett Universal II formula and an 18.5 D IOL was implanted. Postoperatively, the patient's uncorrected visual acuity (UCVA) was 6/18 and best corrected visual acuity (BCVA) was 6/12 with and acceptance of −0.75 DS. Postoperative AL measured using optical biometry was 24.80 mm.

CASE 2

A 48-year-old patient with macula-off RD in right eye was planned for combined cataract surgery with pars plana vitrectomy. The AL measured in right eye using optical biometry (IOLMaster 700) was 15.82 mm with the OCT image showing the detached retina displaced anteriorly. The AL in the fellow eye was 25.47 mm.

The AL measured using contact A-scan was 25.5 mm with a single spike of relatively low amplitude anterior to the scleral spike.

Since the AL obtained on A-scan was comparable to that of fellow eye, the IOL power was calculated using Barrett Universal II formula with an AL value of 25.5 mm and emmetropic target. Postoperatively, the UCVA at 3 months was 6/12 and BSCVA was 6/9 with an acceptance of −0.5 DS.

SECTION 4: Intraocular Lens Power Calculation in Challenging Situations

IOL calculation

OD right		OS left
👁	Eye status	👁
LS: Phakic VS: Vitreous body		LS: Phakic VS: Vitreous body
Ref: --- VA: ---		Ref: --- VA: ---
LVC: Untreated LVC mode: -		LVC: Untreated LVC mode: -
Target ref.: -0.20 D SIA: +0.10 D @ 0°		Target ref.: -0.20 D SIA: +0.10 D @ 0°

Biometric values

OD:
- AL: **15.82 mm (!)**   SD: 9 μm
- ACD: 3.60 mm (!)   SD: 27 μm
- LT: 4.08 mm (!)   SD: 78 μm
- WTW: 12.2 mm
- SE: 40.13 D   SD: 0.02 D   K1: 39.81 D @ 69°
- ΔK: +0.65 D @159°   K2: 40.46 D @159°
- TSE: 40.13 D   SD: 0.01 D   TK1: 39.77 D @ 79°
- ΔTK: +0.72 D @169°   TK2: 40.49 D @169°

OS:
- AL: 25.47 mm   SD: 7 μm
- ACD: 3.47 mm (!)   SD: 16 μm
- LT: 4.04 mm (!)   SD: 81 μm
- WTW: 12.3 mm (!)
- SE: 40.44 D   SD: 0.01 D   K1: 40.00 D @107°
- ΔK: +0.87 D @ 17°   K2: 40.88 D @ 17°
- TSE: 40.49 D   SD: 0.04 D   TK1: 40.01 D @104°
- ΔTK: +0.97 D @ 14°   TK2: 40.98 D @ 14°

TK Alcon AcrySof IQ SN60WF

- Barrett TK Universal II -
LF: +1.88 DF: +5.0

IOL (D)	Ref (D)
+20.00	-0.76
+19.50	-0.39
+19.00	-0.03
+18.50	+0.32
+18.00	+0.67
+18.96	Emmetropia

TK Alcon Clareon CNA0T0

- Barrett TK Universal II -
LF: +2.06 DF: +5.0

IOL (D)	Ref (D)
+20.50	-0.90
+20.00	-0.54
+19.50	-0.18
+19.00	+0.17
+18.50	+0.52
+19.25	Emmetropia

TK Alcon AcrySof Toric SN6AT (2-9)

- Barrett TK Toric -
LF: +1.99 DF: +5.0

	IOL SE	IOL Cyl	IOL axis	Ref SE	Ref Sph	Ref Cyl	Ref Axis
T2	+20.50	+1.00	9°	-0.99	-1.14	+0.31	9°
T2	+20.00	+1.00	9°	-0.62	-0.78	+0.31	9°
T2	+19.50	+1.00	9°	-0.26	-0.42	+0.31	9°
T2	+19.00	+1.00	9°	+0.09	-0.06	+0.31	9°
T2	+18.50	+1.00	9°	+0.44	+0.29	+0.31	9°
	+19.00	+1.41	9°	Emmetropia			

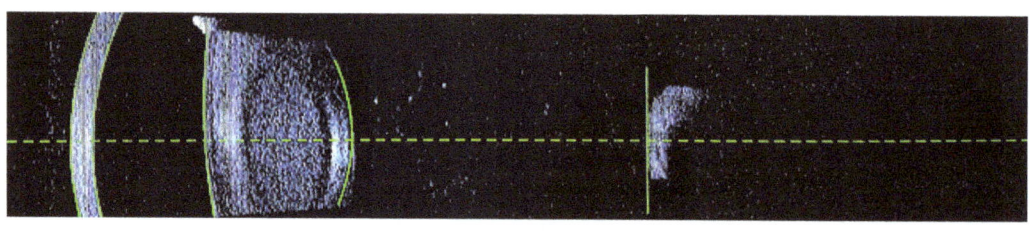

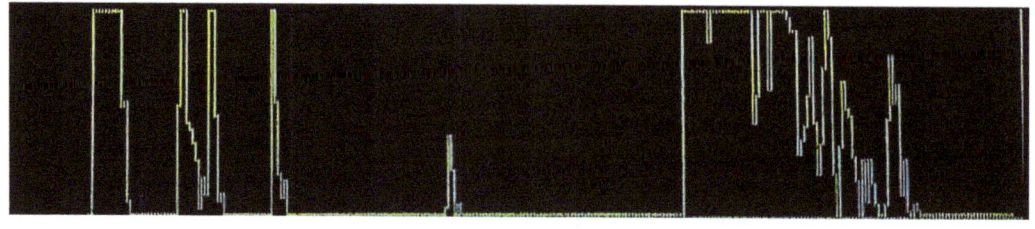

REFERENCES

1. Feng H, Adelman RA. Cataract formation following vitreoretinal procedures. Clin Ophthalmol. 2014;8:1957-65.
2. Wong CW, Ang M, Tsai A, Phua V, Lee SY. A prospective study of biometric stability after scleral buckling surgery. Am J Ophthalmol. 2016;165:47-53.
3. Huang C, Zhang T, Liu J, Ji Q, Tan R. Changes in axial length, central cornea thickness, and anterior chamber depth after rhegmatogenous retinal detachment repair. BMC Ophthalmol. 2016;16:121.
4. Lee DH, Han JW, Kim SS, Byeon SH, Koh HJ, Lee SC, et al. Long-term Effect of scleral encircling on axial elongation. Am J Ophthalmol. 2018;189:139-45.
5. Zhu Z-C, Ke G-J, Wen Y-C, Wu Z-Y. Effects of scleral encircling surgery on vitreous cavity length and diopter. Int J Ophthalmol. 2016;9:572-4.
6. Ophir SS, Friehmann A, Rubowitz A. Circumferential silicone sponge scleral buckling induced axial length changes: case series and comparison to literature. Int J Retina Vitreous. 2017;3:10.
7. Goezinne F, La Heij EC, Berendschot TTJM, Tahzib NG, Cals DWKJ, Liem ATA, et al. Anterior chamber depth is significantly decreased after scleral buckling surgery. Ophthalmology. 2010;117:79-85.
8. Karti O, Selver OB, Ozbek Z, Oner FH, Durak I, Saatci AO. Evaluation of corneal thickness, anterior chamber depth, and iridocorneal angle following scleral buckling surgery with AS-OCT. Ophthalmic Surg Lasers Imaging. 2012;43:S97-102.
9. Cetin E, Ozbek Z, Saatci AO, Durak I. The effect of scleral buckling surgery on corneal astigmatism, corneal thickness, and anterior chamber depth. J Refract Surg. 2006;22:494-9.
10. Okada Y, Nakamura S, Kubo E, Oishi N, Takahashi Y, Akagi Y. Analysis of changes in corneal shape and refraction following scleral buckling surgery. Jpn J Ophthalmol. 2000;44:132-8.
11. Rishi P, Sharma T, Rishi E, Chaudhary SP. Combined scleral buckling and phacoemulsification. Oman J Ophthalmol. 2009;2:15-8.
12. Larkin GB, Flaxel CJ, Leaver PK. Phacoemulsification and silicone oil removal through a single corneal incision. Ophthalmology. 1998;105:2023-7.
13. Krepler K, Mozaffarieh M, Biowski R, Nepp J, Wedrich A. Cataract surgery and silicone oil removal: visual outcome and complications in a combined vs. two step surgical approach. Retina. 2003;23:647-53.
14. Madanagopalan VG, Susvar P, Arthi M. Refractive outcomes of a single-step and a two-step approach for silicone oil removal and cataract surgery. Indian J Ophthalmol. 2019;67:625-9.
15. Murray DC, Durrani OM, Good P, Benson MT, Kirkby GR. Biometry of the silicone oil-filled eye: II. Eye (Lond). 2002;16:727-30.
16. Ghoraba HH, El-Dorghamy AA, Atia AF, Ismail Yassin AE-A. The problems of biometry in combined silicone oil removal and cataract extraction: a clinical trial. Retina. 2002;22:589-96.
17. Suk KK, Smiddy WE, Shi W. Refractive outcomes after silicone oil removal and intraocular lens implantation. Retina. 2013;33:634-41.
18. Nepp J, Krepler K, Jandrasits K, Hauff W, Hanselmayer G, Velikay-Parel M, et al. Biometry and refractive outcome of eyes filled with silicone oil by standardized echography and partial coherence interferometry. Graefes Arch Clin Exp Ophthalmol. 2005;243:967-72.
19. Hoffer KJ. Ultrasound velocities for axial eye length measurement. J Cataract Refract Surg. 1994;20:554-62.
20. Meldrum ML, Aaberg TM, Patel A, Davis J. Cataract extraction after silicone oil repair of retinal detachments due to necrotizing retinitis. Arch Ophthalmol. 1996;114:885-92.
21. Takei K, Sekine Y, Okamoto F, Hommura S. Measurement of axial length of eyes with incomplete filling of silicone oil in the vitreous cavity using x ray computed tomography. Br J Ophthalmol. 2002;86:47-50.

22. Patwardhan SD, Azad R, Sharma Y, Chanana B, Tyagi J. Intraoperative retinoscopy for intraocular lens power estimation in cases of combined phacoemulsification and silicone oil removal. J Cataract Refract Surg. 2009; 35:1190-2.
23. Ianchulev T, Salz J, Hoffer K, Hsu H, Labree L. Intraoperative optical refractive biometry for intraocular lens power estimation without axial length and keratometry measurements. J Cataract Refract Surg. 2005;31:1530-6.
24. Habibabadi HF, Hashemi H, Jalali KH, Amini A, Esfahani MR. Refractive outcome of silicone oil removal and intraocular lens implantation using laser interferometry. Retina. 2005;25:162-6.
25. Grinbaum A, Treister G, Moisseiev J. Predicted and actual refraction after intraocular lens implantation in eyes with silicone oil. J Cataract Refract Surg. 1996;22:726-9.
26. McCartney DL, Miller KM, Stark WJ, Guyton DL, Michels RG. Intraocular lens style and refraction in eyes treated with silicone oil. Arch Ophthalmol. 1987;105:1385-7.
27. Liu Y-L, Yang C-M, Huang J-Y, Chen M-S, Hou Y-C. Postoperative hyperopic shift after cataract surgery in silicone oil-filled eyes. Acta Ophthalmol. 2014;92:e334-5.
28. Mehdizadeh M, Nowroozzadeh MH. Postoperative induced myopia in patients with combined vitrectomy and cataract surgery. J Cataract Refract Surg. 2009;35: 798-9; author reply 799.
29. Tranos PG, Allan B, Balidis M, Vakalis A, Asteriades S, Anogeianakis G, et al. Comparison of postoperative refractive outcome in eyes undergoing combined phacovitrectomy vs cataract surgery following vitrectomy. Graefes Arch Clin Exp Ophthalmol. 2020;258:987-93.
30. Vounotrypidis E, Haralanova V, Muth DR, Wertheimer C, Shajari M, Wolf A, et al. Accuracy of SS-OCT biometry compared with partial coherence interferometry biometry for combined phacovitrectomy with internal limiting membrane peeling. J Cataract Refract Surg. 2019;45:48-53.
31. Jeoung JW, Chung H, Yu HG. Factors influencing refractive outcomes after combined phacoemulsification and pars plana vitrectomy: results of a prospective study. J Cataract Refract Surg. 2007;33: 108-14.
32. Cho KH, Park IW, Kwon SI. Changes in postoperative refractive outcomes following combined phacoemulsification and pars plana vitrectomy for rhegmatogenous retinal detachment. Am J Ophthalmol. 2014; 158:251-6.e2.
33. Jee D, Park Y-R, Jung KI, Kim E, La TY. Refractive errors in high myopic eyes after phacovitrectomy for macular hole. Int J Ophthalmol. 2015;8:369-73.
34. Falkner-Radler CI, Benesch T, Binder S. Accuracy of preoperative biometry in vitrectomy combined with cataract surgery for patients with epiretinal membranes and macular holes: results of a prospective controlled clinical trial. J Cataract Refract Surg. 2008;34:1754-60.
35. Patel D, Rahman R, Kumarasamy M. Accuracy of intraocular lens power estimation in eyes having phacovitrectomy for macular holes. J Cataract Refract Surg. 2007;33:1760-2.
36. Hwang HS, Jee D. Effects of the intraocular lens type on refractive error following phacovitrectomy with gas tamponade. Curr Eye Res. 2011;36:1148-52.
37. Hötte GJ, de Bruyn DP, de Hoog J. Postoperative refractive prediction error after phacovitrectomy: a retrospective study. Ophthalmol Ther. 2018;7:83-94.
38. Sun HJ, Choi KS. Improving intraocular lens power prediction in combined phacoemulsification and vitrectomy in eyes with macular oedema. Acta Ophthalmol 2011;89:575-8.
39. Kim M, Kim HE, Lee DH, Koh HJ, Lee SC, Kim SS. Intraocular Lens Power Estimation in Combined Phacoemulsification and Pars Plana Vitrectomy in Eyes with Epiretinal Membranes: A Case-Control Study. Yonsei Med J. 2015;56:805-11.
40. Vounotrypidis E, Shajari M, Muth DR, Hirnschall N, Findl O, Priglinger S, et al. Refractive outcomes of 8 biometric formulas in combined phacovitrectomy with internal limiting membrane peeling for epiretinal

membrane. J Cataract Refract Surg. 2020;46: 591-7.
41. Ercan ZE, Akkoyun İ, Yaman Pınarcı E, Yılmaz G, Topçu H. Refractive outcome comparison between vitreomacular interface disorders after phacovitrectomy. J Cataract Refract Surg. 2017;43:1068-71.
42. Hirnschall N, Amir-Asgari S, Maedel S, Findl O. Predicting the postoperative intraocular lens position using continuous intraoperative optical coherence tomography measurements. Invest Ophthalmol Vis Sci. 2013;54:5196-203.
43. Manvikar SR, Allen D, Steel DHW. Optical biometry in combined phacovitrectomy. J Cataract Refract Surg. 2009;35:64-9.
44. Abou-Shousha M, Helaly HA, Osman IM. The accuracy of axial length measurements in cases of macula-off retinal detachment. Can J Ophthalmol. 2016;51:108-12.
45. Rahman R, Bong CX, Stephenson J. Accuracy of intraocular lens power estimation in eyes having phacovitrectomy for rhegmatogenous retinal detachment. Retina. 2014;34:1415-20.
46. Pongsachareonnont P, Tangjanyatam S. Accuracy of axial length measurements obtained by optical biometry and acoustic biometry in rhegmatogenous retinal detachment: a prospective study. Clin Ophthalmol. 2018;12:973-80.
47. Kang T-S, Park H-J, Jo Y-J, Kim J-Y. Long-term reproducibility of axial length after combined phacovitrectomy in macula-sparing rhegmatogenous retinal detachment. Sci Rep 2018;8:15856.
48. Rahman R, Kolb S, Bong CX, Stephenson J. Accuracy of user-adjusted axial length measurements with optical biometry in eyes having combined phacovitrectomy for macular-off rhegmatogenous retinal detachment. J Cataract Refract Surg. 2016;42:1009-14.
49. Lee NY, Park SH, Joo CK. Refractive outcomes of phacoemulsification and intraocular lens implantation after pars plana vitrectomy. Retina. 2009;29:487-91.
50. Wang J-K, Chang S-W. Refractive results of phacoemulsification in vitrectomized patients. Int Ophthalmol. 2017;37:673-81.

Intraocular Lens Power Calculation in Extremes of Axial Length

CHAPTER 14

■ INTRODUCTION

Intraocular lens (IOL) power calculation is reasonably accurate in eyes with average *axial length (AL)* of 22–24.5 mm, even with the use of older theoretical or regression-based formulae. The accuracy declines with extremes of AL <22 mm or >26 mm, which may primarily be attributed to difficulty in accurately calculating the effective lens position (ELP), which correlates with AL. The older theoretical formulae used a constant value for ELP, leading to its underestimation in longer eyes with hyperopic predictive error, and overestimation in shorter eyes, resulting in a myopic predictive error.[1] SRK II formula attempted to mitigate this error by modifying the value of A constant based on the AL. The third-generation formulae moved a step further in this direction and incorporate both AL and keratometry (K) in a thin-lens formula to estimate the ELP. In this chapter, we discuss the challenges in calculating IOL power in eyes with extremes of axial lengths, as well as the formulae best suited for such eyes.

■ INTRAOCULAR LENS POWER CALCULATION IN SHORT EYES

Intraocular lens power calculation in short eyes with AL <22 mm remains one of the biggest challenges for a cataract surgeon, with poorer predictability compared to average or longer eyes that worsens in proportion to the decreasing AL.

Sources of Error in Short Eyes

Factors that hinder accurate IOL power calculation in short eyes include anatomical factors, inaccurate biometry and ELP estimation, and IOL-related factors.

- *Anatomical factors:* Shorter eyes have corresponding shorter distance between the IOL and retina, shallow anterior chamber (AC) or steeper K which could contribute to inaccurate IOL power prediction. Conversely, the anterior segment dimensions in these eyes may be normal and thus not proportional to the axial length, an assumption made by the older formulae.[2]
- *High powered IOL:* A high powered thicker lens is usually required in these eyes, which further exaggerates the errors in ELP prediction. Olsen observed a 0.25-mm error in ELP estimation to correspond to a 0.5 D error in a 20-mm eye, as opposed to 0.1 D error in a 30-mm eye.[3]
- *Inaccurate biometry:* An important aspect of IOL power calculation in shorter eyes is the accuracy of AL measurement, as even a small error will result in large refractive error. Thus, optical biometry methods should be preferred over ultrasonic

methods whenever feasible to minimize such errors.[4,5]

- *Other IOL-related factors:* Higher powered IOLs are available in 1 D increments rather than 0.5 D, thus limiting the possibility of achieving emmetropia.[6] An important role could also be played by the IOL power tolerance from the nominal power, which is higher at ±1 D for powers greater than 30 D, as compared to ± 0.4 D for the IOL power range of 15–25 D. Therefore, higher powered IOLs may stray farther from their labeled powers.[7,8]

Choosing the Appropriate Formula in Short Eyes

Most IOL power calculation formulae produce a myopic predictive error in short eyes. Among the third-generation formula, Hoffer Q formula has been classically recommended for the short eyes.[2,9] The less accurate results of SRK-T formula in short eyes may be owing to its basic assumption that the distance from the principal plane of the cornea to the IOL plane is influenced by the axial length. This assumption could be erroneous, as a significant proportion of small eyes have normal anterior chamber anatomy in the pseudophakic state.[7]

Among the fourth-generation formulae, the Haigis and Holladay 2 were found to be better than or comparable to Hoffer Q formula in short eyes.[6] A meta-analysis by Wang et al. reported Haigis to be superior to the third-generation formulae in short eyes.[10] Unlike the third-generation formulae which predict the ELP solely based on the AL and K, Haigis and Holladay 2 formulae use the actual preoperative anterior chamber depth (ACD) without relying on any assumptions for its estimation.[11] The Holladay 2 additionally includes factors such as horizontal corneal diameter, preoperative refraction, and lens thickness for calculating the IOL power, and may be advantageous over the Hoffer Q formula in eyes with <18 mm AL.[7,12]

The choice of formula in short eyes with shallow AC remains controversial. While some authors report Haigis formula to be more accurate than Hoffer Q in eyes with ACD <2.4 mm, others reported contrariwise.[13,14] The reliance of Hoffer Q on AL to estimate the ACD could lead to its underestimation in short eyes with a normal ACD.[10] Likewise, the use of preoperative ACD to estimate the ELP by Haigis formula may be a source of error in shorter eyes showing a significant change in ACD after cataract surgery. The accuracy of a formula in short eyes may, therefore, be determined by multiple factors pertaining to the preoperative ACD, including its relationship to AL, as well as the change in ACD observed after surgery.

Recent studies report the Kane formula to be most accurate in short eyes, with EVO 2.0, Olsen, and Hill RBF formulae also showing good accuracy.[15-17] Kane and EVO 2.0 formulae have been reported to produce most accurate results in eyes requiring IOL power >30 D.[8] Melles et al. reported that Barrett Universal II performed better than third-generation formulae, Haigis, Holladay 2, and Olsen formula in short eyes.[18] Recently introduced formulae such as Zeiss AI Calculator, K6, Pearl-DGS, and Hoffer QST formulae are also promising in short eyes.[19-21]

Intraocular lens constant optimization based on the patient's AL, over and above the individual surgeon-based adjustment is recommended to further reduce the IOL power predictive error in short eyes.[2,11] **Flowchart 1** details the considerations to be taken into account while performing IOL power calculation in short eyes. Despite improvements in IOL formulas, there is a

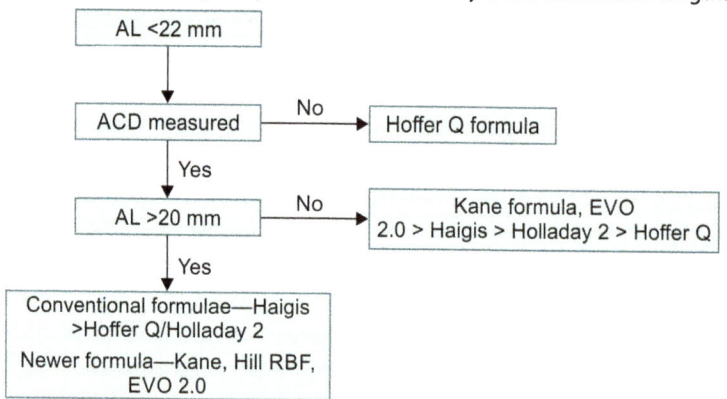

Flowchart 1: Planning IOL power calculation in eyes with short axial lengths

Note:
- *Kane formula:* Requires AL, K, ACD, LT (optional), CCT (optional)
- *Holladay 2:* Requires AL, K, ACD, LT, WTW, age, preoperative refraction (optional)
- *Hill-RBF:* Requires AL, K, ACD, WTW, LT, CCT

(AL: axial length; ACD: anterior chamber depth; CCT: central corneal thickness; IOL: intraocular lens; K: keratometry; LT: lens thickness; WTW: white-to-white)

considerable scope for improvement in accuracy in short eyes. The percentage of eyes within a prediction error of 0.50 D even with the newer formulae range from 43 to 82.3% only.[16]

INTRAOCULAR LENS POWER CALCULATION IN LONG EYES (AL >26 MM)

Intraocular lens power calculation in longer eyes (AL >26 mm) is a more frequently faced challenge by cataract surgeons owing to the increasing prevalence of myopia.

Sources of Error in Long Eyes

Anatomical variations, inaccurate biometry, and IOL design-related factors contribute to errors in IOL power calculation in long eyes.
- *Anatomical factors:* High myopic eyes often have flatter corneas, deeper ACDs, and thinner crystalline lens that may not conform with the assumptions made by the conventional formulae.
- *Inaccurate biometry:* Optical biometry is recommended in longer eyes as ultrasonic biometry could result in erroneous measurements in the presence of a posterior staphyloma, commonly observed with AL >28 mm. Poor fixation due to posterior segment pathology is another factor which could contribute to erroneous biometry.
- *IOL design-related factors:* The IOL design is altered from symmetrically biconvex to meniscus shaped when the power transitions between plus and minus power, i.e., the lower powered (<6 D), zero- and negative-powered IOLs. Thus, in eyes with AL >30 mm where such IOL powers are usually required, position of principal planes lies farther from the geometrical plane of IOL and switches side with the change in IOL power sign. The position of principal planes is related to the ELP and should be accounted for in the A-constant of the formula used, which would be different for negative- and

positive-powered IOLs. The use of constants meant for positive-power IOLs in a negative power IOL would result in a hyperopic predictive error as it would choose an excessively strong minus lens.[22,23]

Choosing the Appropriate Formula in Long Eyes

Among the third-generation formulae, Holladay 1 is traditionally recommended for medium-long eyes (AL = 24.5–26 mm) while SRK T is recommended for AL >26.0 mm.[9] A significant hyperopic surprise, which increases in proportion to the AL (about 0.7–1.5 D), has been observed with the use of standard third-generation formula in longer eyes, with the least hyperopic predictive error noted with SRK-T formula.[24,25] The Haigis formula has performed very well in long eyes and has been found to be more accurate than SRK-T and Holladay 2. Barrett Universal II formula has performed consistently well in long eyes with numerous studies reporting it to be the most accurate in these eyes. While outcomes of Haigis formula are somewhat comparable to Barrett Universal II in eyes with an AL up to 30 mm, the latter is more accurate in eyes with AL >30 mm.[26,27]

To prevent hyperopic predictive errors seen with the use of third- and fourth-generation formulae in myopic eyes, the Wang-Koch (W-K) AL-adjusted formula, based on regression analysis, was suggested for Haigis, Hoffer Q, Holladay 1, SRK/T, and Holladay 2 formula.[28] Though W-K adjustment reduced the hyperopic predictive error observed with these formulae, some authors have reported it to be overly aggressive, resulting in an overshoot leading to myopic outcomes.[18,29] Modified W-K adjustment has been proposed as a less aggressive alternative with a lower myopic predictive error.[29]

The original W-K adjustment may be better suited for extremely long eyes where the risk of hyperopic outcomes is higher.

The newer formula such as Hill-RBF version 2.0, EVO 2.0, Kane formula, and Olsen formula have performed quite well with longer eyes.[18,30] The more consistent results seen with Barrett Universal II, Hill-RBF, or Olsen in long eyes as compared to SRK-T or Haigis may partly be explained by the minimal effect of keratometry on the performance of the former. Conversely, keratometry significantly can affect the accuracy of SRK-T and Haigis formula wherein a steeper K-reading has been associated with a more myopic predictive error with SRK-T, and the reverse with Haigis formula.[18,27]

Intraocular lens power calculation is particularly challenging in the extremely long eyes (AL >30 mm) and those requiring lower (<6 D) or negative IOL powers. Following are the methods proposed for improving accuracy in these patients:

- The use of separate optimized constants for the plus and minus powered IOLs (available on ULIB) is recommended for eyes requiring low or negative powered IOLs, owing to the IOL design related hyperopic predictive error.[23]
- The Barrett Universal II formula, a theoretical formula based on Gaussian thick lens equation, takes into account the position of principal planes of refraction and lens thickness and is known to produce most accurate results in extremely high myopic eyes.
- The Olsen formula, a ray tracing thick lens formula, has been reported to produce outcomes comparable to Barrett Universal II formula in eyes with AL >30 mm.[26]
- The original W-K AL adjustment for Haigis and Holladay 1 formula has been reported

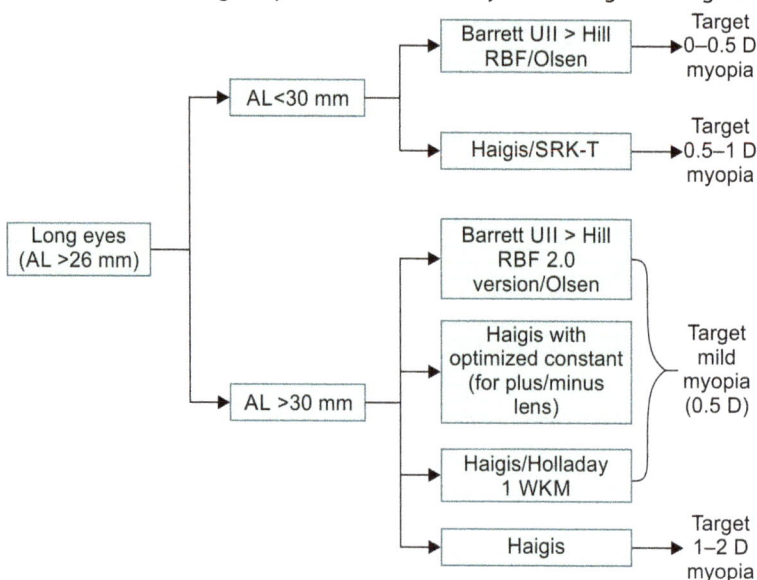

Flowchart 2: Planning IOL power calculation in eyes with long axial lengths

Note:
- *SRK-T, Holladay 1:* Requires AL, K
- *Barrett II Universal:* Requires AL, K, ACD, LT (optional), WTW (optional)
- *Haigis:* Requires AL, K, ACD
- *Hill-RBF:* Requires AL, K, ACD, WTW, LT, CCT
- *Olsen:* Requires AL, K, ACD, LT (optional), CCT (optional)

(AL: axial length; ACD: anterior chamber depth; CCT: central corneal thickness; IOL: intraocular lens; K: keratometry; LT: lens thickness; WTW: white-to-white)

to produce good outcomes in extremely myopic eyes requiring IOL Power < 6 D.[22,25]

- The newer Hill-RBF version 2.0 is modified based on an expanded database with the addition of very short (up to +30 D IOL) and long eyes (meniscus IOLs up to –5 D), with a significant increase in the range of in-bound calculations. The spectrum of the ALs included in this newer version ranges from 20.25 to 37.95 mm, as compared to 20.43–30.15 mm in Version 1, and has been found to perform well in extremely long eyes.

In myopic patients undergoing bilateral surgery, targeting a mild myopic error of about 0.5–1 D is usually sufficient **(Flowchart 2)**. Some authors have suggested preserving a postoperative myopic error of about 2–3 D in myopic patients. Targeting such a substantial myopic error may be prudent in patients undergoing unilateral cataract surgery, taking into account the myopic error in the other eye. It also suits a near-sighted lifestyle and helps avoid any hyperopic refractive surprise, which can be problematic in these patients.[31]

The refractive outcomes in long eyes is somewhat better than short eyes, with 57–86.5% of eyes within a prediction error of 0.50 D.[16]

■ CONCLUSION

Intraocular lens power calculation in eyes with extremes of AL is challenging. Shorter eyes are the most problematic due to higher unpredictability seen even with the newer formulae. Errors in AL measurement or ELP estimation in the longer eyes are minimized by the lower dioptric power of their IOLs, while the reverse is true for the shorter eyes. Accurate biometry is extremely important in short or long eyes and should be performed using optical biometry. Among the older formulae, Haigis, Hoffer Q, and Holladay 2 perform well in the shorter eyes. Newer formulae such as Kane formula, Hill RBF and EVO 2.0 formulae have produced more accurate outcomes.[8,32] For long eyes, Haigis remains a good option among the traditional open access formulae. Barrett Universal II formula has consistently performed well in these eyes. Other newer formulae such as Olsen and Hill RBF also perform very well in these eyes.

CLINICAL CASE EXAMPLES

CASE 1

A 60-year-old male patient was planned for cataract surgery in the left eye. The ocular biometry measured using IOLMaster 700 was as follows:

Parameter	OD	OS
Axial length	19.09 mm	19.06 mm
Keratometry	44.36 D/49.12 D × 1°	43.68 D/ 48.87 D × 177°
Anterior chamber (AC) depth	2.69 mm	2.52 mm
Lens thickness	5.14 mm	5.08 mm
White-to-white (WTW)	11.4 mm	11.2 mm

The IOL power in the left eye calculated using Haigis formula was 37 D/T6.5 Acriol EC toric IOL (177° axis) with a target spherical equivalent of –0.05 D. Postoperative UCVA at 1 month was 6/9 P that improved to 6/9 with an acceptance of –0.25 DS.

CASE 2

A 49-year-old male patient was planned for cataract surgery in the right eye. The ocular biometry measured using IOLMaster 700 was as follows:

Parameter	OD	OS
Axial length	30.07 mm	27.88 mm
Keratometry	41.3 D/42.6 D × 147°	40.94 D/ 42.08 D × 6°
Anterior chamber (AC) Depth	3.63 mm	3.85 mm
Lens thickness	4.08 mm	3.84 mm
White-to-white (WTW)	12.2 mm	12.4 mm

The intraocular lens (IOL) power in the right eye calculated using Barrett Universal II (TK) formula was 6D/T4 (Alcon AcrSof IQ Toric IOL; SN6AT) to be implanted at 148° axis with a target spherical equivalent of –0.30D. Postoperative UCVA at 1 month was 6/6.

REFERENCES

1. Olsen T, Thim K, Corydon L. Accuracy of the newer generation intraocular lens power calculation formulas in long and short eyes. J Cataract Refract Surg 1991;17:187-93.
2. Gavin EA, Hammond CJ. Intraocular lens power calculation in short eyes. Eye (Lond). 2008;22:935-8.
3. Olsen T. Calculation of intraocular lens power: a review. Acta Ophthalmol Scand. 2007;85:472-85.
4. Hoffer KJ, Savini G. IOL Power Calculation in Short and Long Eyes. Asia Pac J Ophthalmol (Phila). 2017;6:330-1.
5. Hoffman RS, Vasavada AR, Allen QB, Snyder ME, Devgan U, Braga-Mele R. Cataract

surgery in the small eye. J Cataract Refract Surg. 2015;41:2565-75.
6. Gökce SE, Zeiter JH, Weikert MP, Koch DD, Hill W, Wang L. Intraocular lens power calculations in short eyes using 7 formulas. J Cataract Refract Surg. 2017;43:892-7.
7. Carifi G, Aiello F, Zygoura V, Kopsachilis N, Maurino V. Accuracy of the refractive prediction determined by multiple currently available intraocular lens power calculation formulas in small eyes. Am J Ophthalmol. 2015;159:577-83.
8. Kane JX, Melles RB. Intraocular lens formula comparison in axial hyperopia with a high-power intraocular lens of 30 or more diopters. J Cataract Refract Surg. 2020;46:1236-9.
9. Aristodemou P, Knox Cartwright NE, Sparrow JM, Johnston RL. Formula choice: Hoffer Q, Holladay 1, or SRK/T and refractive outcomes in 8108 eyes after cataract surgery with biometry by partial coherence interferometry. J Cataract Refract Surg. 2011;37:63-71.
10. Wang Q, Jiang W, Lin T, Wu X, Lin H, Chen W. Meta-analysis of accuracy of intraocular lens power calculation formulas in short eyes. Clin Experiment Ophthalmol. 2018;46:356-63.
11. Day AC, Foster PJ, Stevens JD. Accuracy of intraocular lens power calculations in eyes with axial length <22.00 mm. Clin Exp Ophthalmol. 2012;40:855-62.
12. Hoffer KJ. Clinical results using the Holladay 2 intraocular lens power formula. J Cataract Refract Surg. 2000;26:1233-7.
13. Eom Y, Kang S-Y, Song JS, Kim YY, Kim HM. Comparison of Hoffer Q and Haigis formulae for intraocular lens power calculation according to the anterior chamber depth in short eyes. Am J Ophthalmol. 2014;157:818-824.e2.
14. Yang S, Whang W-J, Joo C-K. Effect of anterior chamber depth on the choice of intraocular lens calculation formula. PLoS One. 2017;12.e0189868.
15. Darcy K, Gunn D, Tavassoli S, Sparrow J, Kane JX. Assessment of the accuracy of new and updated intraocular lens power calculation formulas in 10930 eyes from the UK National Health Service. J Cataract Refract Surg. 2020;46:2-7.
16. Kane JX, Chang DF. Intraocular lens power formulas, biometry, and intraoperative aberrometry: A review. Ophthalmology. 2021;128:e94-114.
17. Chung J, Bu JJ, Afshari NA. Advancements in intraocular lens power calculation formulas. Curr Opin Ophthalmol. 2022;33:35-40.
18. Melles RB, Holladay JT, Chang WJ. Accuracy of intraocular lens calculation formulas. Ophthalmology. 2018;125:169-78.
19. Kenny PI, Kozhaya K, Truong P, Weikert MP, Wang L, Hill WE, et al. Efficacy of segmented axial length and artificial intelligence approaches to intraocular lens power calculation in short eyes. J Cataract Refract Surg. 2023;49:697-703.
20. Shammas HJ, Taroni L, Pellegrini M, Shammas MC, Jivrajka RV. Accuracy of newer intraocular lens power formulas in short and long eyes using sum-of-segments biometry. J Cataract Refract Surg. 2022;48:1113-20.
21. Luo Y, Li H, Gao L, Du J, Chen W, Gao Y, et al. Comparing the accuracy of new intraocular lens power calculation formulae in short eyes after cataract surgery: a systematic review and meta-analysis. Int Ophthalmol. 2022;42:1939-56.
22. Abulafia A, Barrett GD, Rotenberg M, et al. Intraocular lens power calculation for eyes with an axial length greater than 26.0 mm: Comparison of formulas and methods. J Cataract Refract Surg. 2015;41:548-56.
23. Haigis W. Intraocular lens calculation in extreme myopia. J Cataract Refract Surg. 2009;35:906-11.
24. Ji J, Liu Y, Zhang J, Wu X, Shao W, Ma B, et al. Comparison of six methods for the intraocular lens power calculation in high myopic eyes. Eur J Ophthalmol. 2021;31:96-102.
25. Geggel HS. Comparison of formulas and methods for high myopia patients requiring intraocular lens powers less than six diopters. Int Ophthalmol. 2018;38:1497-504.
26. Rong X, He W, Zhu Q, Qian D, Lu Y, Zhu X. Intraocular lens power calculation in eyes

with extreme myopia: Comparison of Barrett Universal II, Haigis, and Olsen formulas. J Cataract Refract Surg. 2019;45:732-7.
27. Wan KH, Lam TCH, Yu MCY, Chan TCY. Accuracy and precision of intraocular lens calculations using the new Hill-RBF Version 2.0 in eyes with high axial myopia. Am J Ophthalmol. 2019;205:66-73.
28. Wang L, Shirayama M, Ma XJ, Kohnen T, Koch DD Optimizing intraocular lens power calculations in eyes with axial lengths above 25.0 mm. Cataract Refract Surg. 2011;37:2018-27.
29. Liu J, Wang L, Chai F, Han Y, Qian S, Koch DD, et al. Comparison of intraocular lens power calculation formulas in Chinese eyes with axial myopia. J Cataract Refract Surg. 2019;45:725-31.
30. Ma Y, Xiong R, Liu Z, Young CA, Wu Y, Zheng D, et al. Network meta-analysis of IOL power calculation formula accuracy in 1,016 eyes with long axial length. Am J Ophthalmol. 2023:S0002-9394(23)00375-6.
31. Chen C, Xu X, Miao Y, Zheng G, Sun Y, Xu X. Accuracy of intraocular lens power formulas involving 148 eyes with long axial lengths: a retrospective chart-review study. J Ophthalmol. 2015;2015:976847.
32. Kane JX, Van Heerden A, Atik A, Petsoglou C. Accuracy of 3 new methods for intraocular lens power selection. J Cataract Refract Surg. 2017;43:333-9.

CHAPTER 15

Intraocular Lens Power of Piggyback IOLs and Secondary IOLs

■ INTRODUCTION

Primary in-the-bag implantation of an intraocular lens (IOL), though desirable, may not always be possible due to preoperative factors or intraoperative complications during cataract surgery. Depending on the anatomical factors, the secondary IOL may need to be implanted in the ciliary sulcus, fixed to the sclera or iris, or placed in the anterior chamber angle. Moreover, piggyback or supplemental IOL implantation involves placing an additional IOL in a pseudophakic patient to treat residual refractive error. Standard formulae calculate IOL power for in-the-bag implantation, and the power for secondary IOLs need to be adjusted based on the displacement from this location, as a 1-mm displacement of a 21 D IOL may induce a 1.4 D refractive error.[1,2] In this chapter, we describe IOL power calculation methods for secondary IOL implantation along with their outcomes.

■ ANGLE-SUPPORTED ANTERIOR CHAMBER INTRAOCULAR LENS

Selection of an appropriate angle-supported anterior chamber IOL (ACIOL) should take into account two important parameters—IOL size and power. Haptic-to-haptic diameter of an ACIOL should be 1 mm more than the horizontal white-to-white corneal diameter. While the exact IOL power is determined by the respective A-constant of the IOL, a rough estimation of the required IOL power may be obtained by subtracting 3 D from the spherical power of the calculated in-the-bag IOL power. The manufacturer-recommended A-constants for the various open loop ACIOLs are listed in **Table 1**. The IOL sizing based on white-to-white corneal diameter

TABLE 1: Angle-supported ACIOLs along with their A-constants and sizes

ACIOL	A-constant	Available sizes
Kelman Multiflex III (Alcon Laboratories, Fort Worth, Texas, USA)	115.54 (optical) 115.3 (ultrasound)	12, 12.5, 13, 13.5, 14, 14.5 mm
122UV ACIOL (Bausch and Lomb Inc., New York, USA)	116.14 (optical) 115.8 (ultrasound)	12.5, 13.75 mm
Aurolens ACIOL (Aurolab, India)	115.3	12, 12.5, 13 mm
Liberty Lens: 302 L (Appasamy Associates Private Limited, India)	115.3	12.5 mm
OPAB ACIOL (Hanita Lenses, Israel)	114.9	13 mm

(ACIOL: anterior chamber intraocular lens)

as recommended by the manufacturers is detailed in **Table 2**.

Outcomes: Studies reveal good refractive outcomes with ACIOL placement with 40.4–65.5% eyes achieving a spherical equivalent within ±0.5 D of target.[3,4]

IRIS-FIXATED INTRAOCULAR LENS

Iris fixation of IOLs in aphakia can be either performed by suturing three-piece IOLs to the iris or by enclavation of iris-claw lenses anterior to iris or in the retropupillary space. Iris-fixated IOLs have more accurate refractive outcomes as compared to scleral-fixated IOLs (SFIOLs), owing to better predictability of effective lens position (ELP) and standardized IOL power calculation formulae.

The SRK-T formula is most commonly used for IOL power calculation of iris-claw lenses. At present, there is a dearth of literature on the outcomes of newer formulae such as Barrett Universal II in these cases. The lack of feasibility of the newer formulae may be attributed to implantation of these IOLs in aphakic eyes or those with IOL dislocation.[5] Care should be taken to use a different A-constant when calculating the power of the iris-fixated IOL **(Table 3)**. The Artisan® aphakia IOL (Ophtec, Groeningen, The Netherlands) and Verisyse® IOL for aphakia (model VRS54, Abbott Laboratories, Santa Clara, US) are most commonly used. The manufacturer-provided A-constants with SRK/T formula for these lenses are 115.0 (ultrasound) and 115.7 (optical biometry) for anterior fixation and 116.8 (ultrasound), and 116.9 (optical biometry) for retropupillary fixation.[6]

Outcomes: Retropupillary implantation of iris-claw lenses results in 60–80% of cases

TABLE 2: ACIOL sizing based on white-to-white corneal diameter as recommended by manufacturers

Alcon ACIOL		
WTW (mm)	IOL diameter (mm)	Model
11.0–11.4	12.0	MTA2UO
11.5–11.9	12.5	MTA3UO
12.0–12.4	13	MTA4UO
12.5–12.9	13.5	MTA5UO
13.0–13.4	14	MTA6UO
13.5–13.9	14.5	MTA7UO
Bausch and Lomb ACIOL		
WTW (mm)	IOL diameter (mm)	Model
10.0–11.49	12.5	S122UV
11.5–12.25	13.75	L122UV

(ACIOL: anterior chamber intraocular lens; IOL: intraocular lens; WTW: white-to-white)

TABLE 3: Iris-claw lenses along with their manufacturer-recommended A-constants for pre-pupillary and retropupillary fixation

Iris-claw intraocular lens	A-constant (anterior fixation)	A-constant (retropupillary fixation)
Verisyse IOL for aphakia (VRSA54, Abbott Laboratories, Inc., Abbott Park, IL, USA)	115	116.9
Artisan Aphakia (Ophtec, Groningen, The Netherlands)	115	116.9
Excelens (Excel Optics Pvt. Ltd., Chennai, India)	115	117.2
Freedom (Freedom Ophthalmic Pvt. Ltd., Hosur, India)	115	117.4
Optima (Rainbow Meditech LLC, Chennai, India)	115.7	117.2
OV lens (Care Group, India)	114.9	117.2

with spherical equivalent within ±1.00 D of target.[5,6] With pre-pupillary enclavation, nearly 85–100% of cases achieve a spherical equivalent within ±1.00 D.[6,7]

SCLERAL-FIXATED INTRAOCULAR LENS

Intraocular lens power adjustments for SFIOLs remain a challenge owing to the variability in the anatomical position of IOL, which is primarily determined by the location of sutures or how far from the limbus the haptics are externalized. A more hyperopic shift is seen when the haptic is fixated more posteriorly.[8] In addition, IOL design and technique of IOL fixation (sutured or intrasclerally fixated) may also influence the refractive outcomes. A three-piece IOL is typically used for intrascleral fixation and a single-piece IOL for sutured scleral fixation. The haptics of three-piece IOLs are at an angle with the optic that can impact the optic vault. Meanwhile, in sutured SFIOL, the suture tension can impact the IOL position with more lax sutures resulting in a posterior displacement and vice versa.[9] Presence of capsular remnants may also impact the final IOL position. Moreover, SFIOLs are prone to slight tilt or decentration, which further makes the refractive outcomes unpredictable.

Most authors have observed a hyperopic outcome with SFIOL implantation on using in-the-bag IOL calculations, and recommend targeting a myopic error ranging from –0.5 to –0.75 D.[9-12]

Interestingly, some studies report a mild myopic shift while using ULIB constants and recommend that surgeons optimize the constants for each formula based on their previous clinical data in order to reduce the postoperative predictive error.[8,13,14]

Among the formulae, third-generation formulae, namely SRK-T and Holladay 1, give the most accurate outcomes, outperforming the newer ones such as Haigis and Barrett Universal II.[13,15,16] A reliable estimation of preoperative anterior chamber depth (ACD) in cases planned for SFIOL implantation is often not possible, which may adversely affect the accuracy of these newer formulae that rely on ACD for estimating ELP.[14]

Outcomes: Refractive outcomes post SFIOL implantation are less accurate than routine capsular bag IOL implantation, with 27.3–64% eyes within ±0.5 D of the predicted spherical equivalent.[17,18]

PIGGYBACK INTRAOCULAR LENSES

The concept of piggyback IOLs was introduced by Gayton et al. in 1993 to manage a case of hyperopia requiring a very high IOL power that exceeded the highest available IOL power. The authors implanted two IOLs within the capsular bag to provide adequate power.[19] The technique was later adapted to treat residual ametropia, myopia, and hyperopia.

The most common indication for piggyback IOL implantation is residual ametropia, especially a hyperopic error, after cataract surgery. Other indications include highly hyperopic or nanophthalmic eyes that primarily require very high IOL powers, which may not be commercially available in a single IOL. More recently, there has been a renewed interest in piggyback IOLs as a technique to provide spectacle independence to patients who already are pseudophakic by implanting a low-power multifocal IOL or toric supplemental IOL. In order to implant a piggyback IOL, the primary IOL should be stable within the capsular bag and the patients should have an adequate AC depth (>3 mm) with a healthy endothelial cell count.

Approach to IOL power calculation depends on whether primary polypseudophakia or secondary polypseudophakia is being considered.

Intraocular Lens Power Calculation in Primary Polypseudophakia

Primary polypseudophakia is performed in cases requiring very high IOL powers beyond the range that are routinely manufactured. One IOL is implanted in the bag and a second IOL in the sulcus. Dr Warren Hill has described the IOL power calculation method in these cases in detail. Firstly, the total IOL power needed at the capsular bag plane is calculated targeting for a slight myopia of about 0.75 D. As these are short eyes, Holladay 2, optimized Haigis, or Hoffer Q formulae can be used. The maximum available IOL power to be implanted in capsular bag is then subtracted from this power. Based on the residual power, the power of the IOL to be implanted in the ciliary sulcus is calculated using appropriate adjustments **(Table 4)**. This adjustment differs from that of an IOL being placed in the ciliary sulcus in an aphakic eye, as the sulcus IOL in primary polypseudophakia is implanted in front of an IOL within the bag giving it a more anterior shift. It is recommended to implant IOLs of different materials within the bag and sulcus, owing to the risk of intra-lenticular opacification when one acrylic IOL is placed over another. An acrylic IOL with a negative shape factor is suitable for capsular bag placement while a large diameter, biconvex silicone IOL may be implanted in the sulcus. Boisvert et al. devised a "Pediatric Piggyback IOL Calculator" to select IOL power combinations for temporary polypseudophakia in children undergoing cataract surgery. They recommend an initial postoperative target of moderate hyperopia, with the anterior IOL having approximately 20% of the total required IOL power for optimal outcomes. The anterior IOL may be removed once the child's myopic error equals half the anterior IOL power.[20]

Intraocular Lens Power Calculation for Secondary Piggyback Intraocular Lens Implantation

Intraocular lens power calculation for a secondary piggyback IOL primarily relies on the postoperative pseudophakic refractive spherical equivalent, piggyback IOL's A-constant and biometry. Gayton et al. proposed using a plus powered piggyback IOL with a power that is 1.5 times the spherical equivalent in a hyperopic surprise and a minus powered IOL equal to the spherical equivalent for correcting a myopic surprise.[21,22] Holladay also recommended a 1-for-1 formula for myopic refractive errors and a 1.5 conversion factor for hyperopic errors.[23] Gills proposed a nomogram for piggyback IOL power calculation based on the type and magnitude of residual error and the axial length as detailed in **Table 5**.[23]

Other more sophisticated approaches include the Hill Refractive Vergence Formula, Holladay R Formula, and Barrett Rx Formula, and may be more accurate in patients with larger residual refractive errors (>7 D).

TABLE 4: Adjustments for power of the IOL to be implanted in the ciliary sulcus based on residual power in primary polypseudophakia

Residual IOL power	Power adjustment for sulcus IOL
+30 D to +25.5 D	Subtract 1.5 D
+25 D to +15.5 D	Subtract 1.0 D
+15 D to +8.5 D	Subtract 0.5 D
+8.0 D to +1 D	No change required

(IOL: intraocular lens)

TABLE 5: Gills' nomogram for piggyback IOL power calculation

Residual hyperopia	
Axial length	IOL power
<22 mm	1.5 × SE + 1
22–25 mm	1.4 × SE + 1
>25 mm	1.3 × SE + 1
Residual myopia	
Axial length	IOL power
<22 mm	1.5 × SE − 1
22–25 mm	1.4 × SE − 1
>25 mm	1.3 × SE − 1

(IOL: intraocular lens; SE: postoperative spherical equivalent)

Refractive vergence formula, introduced by Holladay, uses the residual refraction, vertex distance, keratometry, and a proprietary formula to calculate the required additional power of the piggyback lens. It does not require axial length measurement or the power of pre-existing in-the-bag IOL.[24] It was popularized by Dr Warren Hill who incorporated it into a spreadsheet that can be readily accessed online for IOL power calculation (https://www.doctor-hill.com/physicians/docs/R-verg-Hill.xls). The Holladay R formula is a sophisticated version of the refractive vergence formula and is available commercially on the Holladay IOL Consultant software package (https://www.hicsoap.com). The Barrett Rx formula is derived from the Barrett Universal II formula and is available online (www.apacrs.org). As opposed to refractive vergence formula that uses an IOL-specific value as the basis for the effective lens position (ELP), the Barrett Rx formula back calculates the actual ELP for the given postoperative refractive error, thus allowing it to account for IOLs having different lens constants. The power and model of both the implanted IOL and new IOL model, the postoperative refractive outcome, and patient's ocular biometric data are used to predict the power of the new IOL. In addition to piggyback IOL power calculation, it may also be used for cases of IOL surprise requiring IOL exchange and rotation of toric IOLs from its existing axis.

Intraocular lenses specifically designed for implantation into the ciliary sulcus in pseudophakic patients as add-on lenses include the Sulcoflex IOL (Rayner Intraocular Lenses Ltd, USA), the Add-On IOL (HumanOptics, Germany), first Add-On IOL (1stQ GmbH, Mannheim, Germany) and Sulcofix Add-On IOL (Care Group, India). Online calculators for IOL power calculation of piggyback lenses are available for Sulcoflex IOL (https://www.raytrace.rayner.com/calculations/new?product=Sulcflexnt) and first Q Add-On IOL (https://www.1stq.de/en/addon-calculator), where the surgeon needs to enter the residual refractive error along with biometric data.

Outcomes: Refractive outcomes of piggyback IOL implantation in pseudophakic patients have been very promising with 72–100% of patients achieving outcomes within 0.5 D of target refraction.[25-27]

SULCUS-FIXATED INTRAOCULAR LENS

A reduction in IOL power ranging from 0 to 1.5 D may be required depending on the power of the capsular bag IOL to compensate for the myopic shift induced by sulcus placement. Thicker lens with higher effective power requires higher reduction in power.[28] Before making the adjustments, the surgeon should check if the A-constant of the sulcus IOL is nearly the same as the original IOL, or it needs to be adjusted for as well. In

TABLE 6: IOL power adjustment required for sulcus IOL implantation during cataract surgery

Capsular bag IOL power	Power adjustment for sulcus IOL
0 to +9.0	No change
+9.5 to +18.0	−0.50
+18.5 to +27.0	−1.00
> +27.5	−1.50
Optic capture	No change

(IOL: intraocular lens)

TABLE 7: Sliding scale for IOL power adjustment required for sulcus IOL implantation

Capsular bag IOL power	Power adjustment for sulcus IOL
≥25 D	Subtract 2 D
+20.00 D to <25 D	Subtract 1.5 D
+15.00 D to <20 D	Subtract 1.0 D
+10.00 D to <15 D	Subtract 0.5 D
<10 D	No change required

(IOL: intraocular lens)

case optic capture is performed to place the optic beneath the capsulorhexis, no change in power is required. **Table 6** details the adjustment following "the rule of 9s" required for IOL power correction for unanticipated implantation of IOL in sulcus during cataract surgery.[28,29] Suto et al. provided a sliding scale for sulcus IOL power adjustment based on calculations performed using computer simulation **(Table 7)**.[30] Greater reductions have been recommended for shorter axial length eyes (AL <22 mm).[2,30] Dubey et al. recommended a 0.5 D reduction for IOL powers below 18 D, 1 D reduction for 18–25 D, and 1.5–2 D for IOL power >25 D (the range allows for greater reduction for higher-power planned lenses or shorter ALs).[2]

CONCLUSION

Refractive outcomes of secondary IOL implantation are less predictable as compared to primary in-the-bag implantation, and appropriate correction factors should be applied based on the final effective lens position. Refractive outcomes of iris-fixated and angle-supported ACIOLs are more accurate as compared to scleral-fixated IOLs. Approaches to piggy-back IOL power calculation have become more sophisticated and predictable with the advent of several online platforms to estimate the add-on IOL power based on the patient's residual refractive error and biometry. More recently, premium (toric and multifocal) piggyback or supplemental IOLs have been employed to achieve spectacle independence in pseudophakic patients.[31]

CLINICAL CASE EXAMPLES

CASE 1

A 45-year-old pseudophakic patient presented with an uncorrected visual acuity (UCVA) of 6/60 in right eye and a best spectacle corrected visual acuity of 6/6 and final acceptance of −5 DS. The patient had undergone cataract surgery in right eye 5 months ago and did not possess the records of the IOL that was implanted. The ocular biometry parameters of right eye were as follows:

- *Axial length:* 26 mm
- *Keratometry:* 42.00 D/43.00 D/ at 100°/20°
- *AC depth:* 3.6 mm

The patient was planned for a piggyback IOL (Sulcoflex, Rayner Intraocular Lenses Ltd, USA) implantation and the IOL power was calculated using the online IOL power calculation software provided by the manufacturer (https://www.raytrace.rayner.com/calculations/new?product=Sulcflexnt).

SECTION 4: Intraocular Lens Power Calculation in Challenging Situations

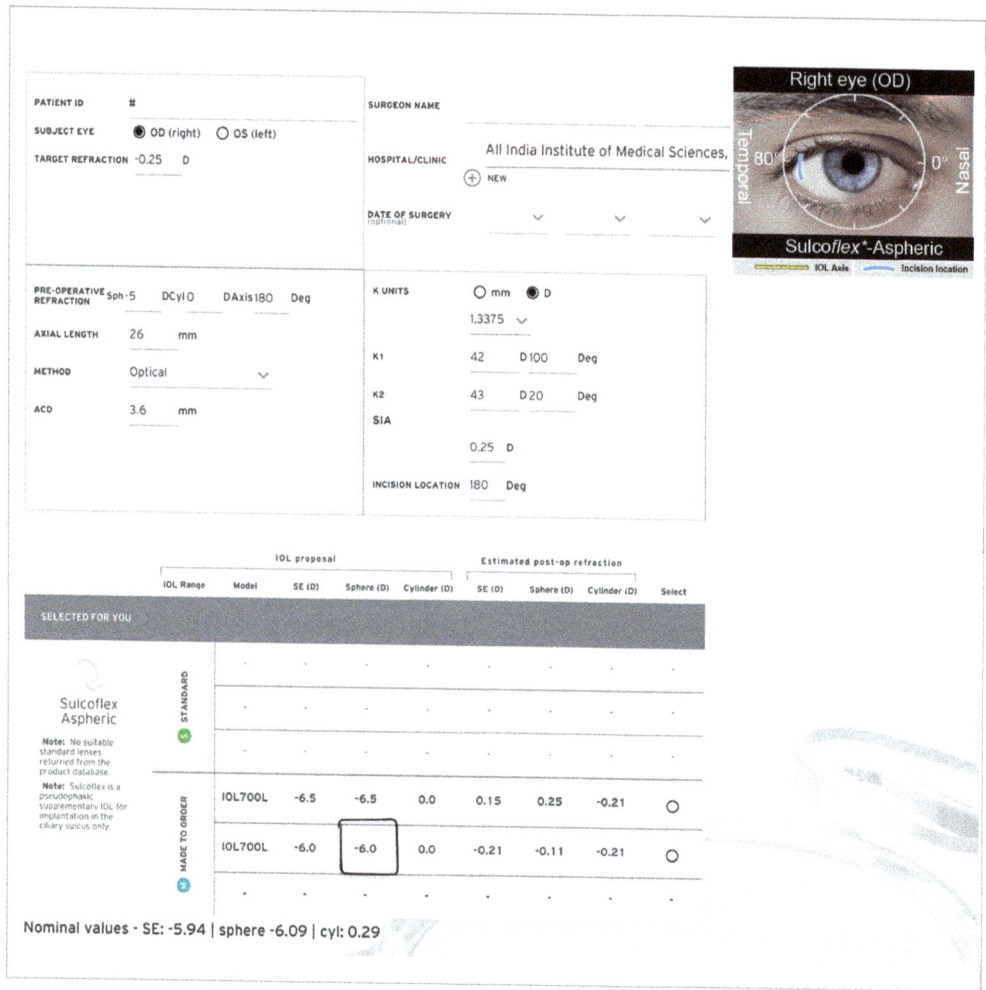

A piggyback IOL of −6.00 D was implanted in the sulcus in the right eye. The postoperative UCVA was 6/6.

■ CASE 2

A 50-year-old pseudophakic patient presented with an UCVA of 6/36 in right eye and a best spectacle corrected visual acuity of 6/6 and final acceptance of −4 DS. The patient had undergone cataract surgery in right eye 5 years ago with an Alcon AcrySof IQ IOL implantation in capsular bag following which he had a UCVA of 6/6. Later on the patient underwent scleral buckling surgery for retinal detachment, following which he developed a myopic refractive error due to axial elongation.

The patient was planned for a piggyback IOL implantation and the IOL power was calculated using the Refractive Vergence Formula described by Holladay (https://www.doctor-hill.com/physicians/docs/R-verg-Hill.xls). The effective lens position (ELPo) of the piggyback IOL was taken as the optimized effective lens position for the capsular bag lens (manufacturer's ACD) reduced by 0.65 mm (i.e., 5.49–0.65).

OL Power Calculations From Refractive Data - Refractive Vergence Formula for Pseudophakic and Aphakic Eyes v. 02.8
Warren E. Hill, MD, FACS   East Valley Ophthalmology, Ltd.   Mesa, Arizona USA

Patient: xxx
Date: xxx
Position: Piggyback IOL
IOL: Staar AQ-5010V
Referring Physician: xxx

Note: Do not enter data into the tan colored boxes

ELPo	Vtx	Kk1	Kk2	Ko - avg	Pre Op Seq	Post Op Rx	IOL Power
4.84	12.0	42.00	43.00	41.98	-4.00	-0.25	-4.88

Staar AQ-5010V three-piece silicone IOL of −5 D was implanted in the sulcus and the patient achieved a UCVA of 6/6 postoperatively.

REFERENCES

1. Giers U, Epple C, Schütte E. [Flattening of the anterior chamber and myopic results in sulcus fixation of posterior chamber lenses]. Klin Monbl Augenheilkd. 1989;195:353-5.
2. Dubey R, Birchall W, Grigg J. Improved refractive outcome for ciliary sulcus-implanted intraocular lenses. Ophthalmology. 2012;119:261-5.
3. Sahoo S, Parida P, Mohanty A, Das S, Mohamed A, Sahu SK. Outcome of four-point fixated open loop polymethyl methacrylate anterior chamber intraocular lens. Int Ophthalmol. 2022;42:1051-9.
4. Gore DM, Wilkins MR. Refractive outcomes in anterior chamber intraocular lenses. Int Ophthalmol. 2013;33:453-4.
5. Drolsum L, Kristianslund O. Implantation of retropupillary iris-claw lenses: a review on surgical management and outcomes. Acta Ophthalmol. 2021;99:826-36.
6. Huerva V, Ascaso FJ, Caral I, Grzybowski A. Calculation of iris-claw IOL power for correction of late in-the-bag IOL complex dislocation. BMC Ophthalmol. 2017;17:122.
7. Hernández Martínez A, Almeida González CV. Iris-claw intraocular lens implantation: Efficiency and safety according to technique. J Cataract Refract Surg. 2018;44:1186-91.
8. Lee R, Govindaraju V, Farley ND, Abbey AM, Stem MS, Shields RA, et al. Refractive outcomes after sutureless intrascleral fixation of intraocular lens with pars plana vitrectomy. Retina 2021;41(4):822-6.
9. Ohr MP, Wisely CE. Refractive outcomes and accuracy of IOL power calculation with the SRK/T formula for sutured, scleral-fixated Akreos AO60 intraocular lenses. Graefes Arch Clin Exp Ophthalmol. 2020;258:2125-9.
10. Aykut V, Esen F, Sali F, Oguz H. Refractive outcome of trocar-assisted sutureless scleral fixation with 3-piece intraocular lenses. Int Ophthalmol. 2021;41:2689-94.
11. Abbey AM, Hussain RM, Shah AR, Faia LF, Wolfe JD, Williams GA. Sutureless scleral fixation of intraocular lenses: outcomes of two approaches. The 2014 Yasuo Tano Memorial Lecture. Graefes Arch Clin Exp Ophthalmol. 2015;253:1-5.
12. McMillin J, Wang L, Wang MY, Al-Mohtaseb Z, Khandelwal S, Weikert M, et al. Accuracy of intraocular lens calculation formulas for flanged intrascleral intraocular lens fixation with double-needle technique. J Cataract Refract Surg. 2021;47:855-8.
13. Schranz M, Reumüller A, Kostolna K, Novotny C, Schartmüller D, Abela-Formanek C. Refractive outcome and lens power calculation after intrascleral intraocular lens fixation: a comparison of three-piece and

one-piece intrascleral fixation technique. Eye Vis (Lond). 2023;10:29.
14. Lian Z, Cao Q, Qi H, Young CA, Zhang X, Jin G, et al. Accuracy of intraocular lens power formulas for eyes with scleral-sutured intraocular lenses in congenital ectopia lentis. J Cataract Refract Surg. 2022;48:469-74.
15. Li Z, Lian Z, Young CA, Zhao J, Jin G, Zheng D. Accuracy of intraocular lens calculation formulas for eyes with insufficient capsular support. Ann Transl Med. 2021;9:324.
16. Botsford BW, Williams AM, Conner IP, Martel JN, Eller AW. Scleral fixation of intraocular lenses with gore-tex suture: refractive outcomes and comparison of lens power formulas. Ophthalmol Retina. 2019;3:468-72.
17. Vaiano AS, Hoffer KJ, Greco A, Greco A, D'Amico G, Pasqualitto V, et al. Accuracy of IOL power calculation using the new carlevale sutureless scleral fixation posterior chamber IOL. J Refract Surg. 2021;37:472-6.
18. Pardini D, Lucatto LF, Junior OM, Maia A, Hammamji K, Dirani A, et al. Outcomes of Pars Plana Vitrectomy and 4-Point Sutured Scleral Fixation of Akreos Ao60 Intraocular Lens in Clinical Settings: a case series. Ophthalmol Retina. 2023;7:59-66.
19. Gayton JL, Sanders VN. Implanting two posterior chamber intraocular lenses in a case of microphthalmos. J Cataract Refract Surg. 1993;19:776-7.
20. Boisvert C, Beverly DT, McClatchey SK. Theoretical strategy for choosing piggyback intraocular lens powers in young children. J AAPOS. 2009;13:555-7.
21. Kieval JZ, Al-Hashimi S, Davidson RS, Hamilton DR, Jackson MA, LaBorwit S, et al. Prevention and management of refractive prediction errors following cataract surgery. J Cataract Refract Surg. 2020;46:1189-97.
22. Gayton JL, Sanders V, Van der Karr M, Raanan MG. Piggybacking intraocular implants to correct pseudophakic refractive error. Ophthalmology. 1999;106:56-9.
23. Shepard D. Consultation section: piggyback intraocular lenses. Ann Ophthalmol. 1998;30: 203-6.
24. Holladay JT. Standardizing constants for ultrasonic biometry, keratometry, and intraocular lens power calculations. J Cataract Refract Surg. 1997;23:1356-70.
25. Gills JP, Fenzl RE. Minus-power intraocular lenses to correct refractive errors in myopic pseudophakia. J Cataract Refract Surg. 1999; 25:1205-8.
26. Basarir B, Kaya V, Altan C, Karakus S, Pinarci EY, Demirok A. The use of a supplemental sulcus fixated IOL (HumanOptics Add-On IOL) to correct pseudophakic refractive errors. Eur J Ophthalmol. 2012;22: 898-903.
27. Venter JA, Oberholster A, Schallhorn SC, Pelouskova M. Piggyback intraocular lens implantation to correct pseudophakic refractive error after segmental multifocal intraocular lens implantation. J Refract Surg. 2014;30:234-9.
28. Mehta R, Aref AA. Intraocular Lens Implantation In The Ciliary Sulcus: Challenges And Risks. Clin Ophthalmol. 2019;13:2317-23.
29. Cheng KKW, Tint NL, Sharp J, Alexander P. Surgical management of aphakia. J Cataract Refract Surg. 2022;48:1453-61.
30. Suto C. Sliding scale of IOL power for sulcus fixation using computer simulation. J Cataract Refract Surg. 2004;30:2452-4.
31. Manzouri B, Dari M, Claoué C. Supplementary IOLs: Monofocal and Multifocal, Their Applications and Limitations. Asia Pac J Ophthalmol (Phila). 2017;6:358-63.

Index

Page numbers followed by *f* refer to figure, *fc* refer to flowchart, and *t* refer to table.

A

Aberrometry-based formulae 68
Ablative corneal refractive surgery 98
Abulafia-Koch formula 50
Actual spherical equivalent 65
Alcon ACIOL 157
Alcon online toric calculator incorporates
    Barrett calculator 51*f*
Angle-supported ACIOLs 156, 156*t*
Anisometropia, possibility of unexpected 116
ANTERION 42, 49
Anterior chamber 136
    depth 6, 30, 36, 37, 39, 62, 69, 70, 86, 122, 130, 134
        personalized 62
        postoperative 58, 93
        preoperative 149, 158
        pseudophakic 61
    intraocular lens 156, 157
    measurement, deepest 11
    shallow 148
Anterior corneal
    astigmatism 48
    curvature measurements 91, 95
    surface 23
        devices measuring 23
    curvature 22, 37, 125*f*
Anterior fixation 157
Anterior radius 70
Anterior segment optical coherence tomography 68
Aphakia 157
Aphakic eye 10
Aphakic pediatric eyes, refractive growth in 112
Aphakic refraction, intraoperative 91, 137
Aramberri double-K method 88
Argos 41, 44
Artificial intelligence 6, 75, 76, 77*t*
    application of 5
    based formulas 5
    fallacies of 79
    machine-learning 76*t*
    methodology and techniques 75
Artisan aphakia 157
Artisan® aphakia intraocular lens 157
A-scan
    biometry measures 9
    ultrasound biometry 13*t*
Aspheric monofocal intraocular lens 128
Atlas topographer 91
Automated intraoperative refraction 136
Automated keratometers 27, 49, 124
Automated positioning system 40
Average central corneal power 30, 98
Axial length 5, 9, 14, 15, 36, 37, 58, 62, 93, 121, 123, 130, 136, 141, 160
    estimation 11*t*
        methods for 136
        optical biometry for 14*t*
    extremes of 71
    intraoperative measurement of 137
    measurement 15, 113
        inaccurate 139

B

Barrett formula 41
Barrett online toric calculator 51*f*
Barrett Rx formula 159
Barrett True-K
    formula 89, 103
    no-history method 94
Barrett universal formula 62, 64, 126, 153
Bausch and Lomb
    ACIOL 157
    keratometer 26
Baylor nomogram 50
Baylor toric intraocular lens nomogram 50*t*
BESSt formula 95
Binkhorst formula 3
    modified 3
Biometric parameter 37*t*, 134
Biometry 5, 7, 33, 113, 123
    accurate 9, 121
    challenges in 127
    changes in 134*t*
    inaccurate 148, 150
    parameters 34*t*
    timing of 123
    ultrasonic 9, 123
    ultrasound 9, 14, 17

C

Calculate corneal power, optical principles to 21*fc*
Capsular bag intraocular lens power 161
Cassini corneal shape analyzer 49

Cataract 135
   surgery 115*t*, 121, 127, 138, 161*t*
      staged 135
Caucasian eyes 79
Central corneal power 91, 93
   anterior 90
Central corneal thickness 37, 70, 140
Charged-couple device camera 39
Ciliary sulcus 159*t*
Circumferential buckles 135
Clayman's formula 3
Colenbrander formula 3
Combined phacovitrectomy procedures 138
Combined tomographers 36
Combined vector-A/B-scan method 142
Contact lens
   in diopters, base curve of 93
   method 38, 91
Contact lens at corneal plane
   spherical equivalent refractive error with 93
   spherical equivalent refractive error without 93
Contact technique 10, 11
Contact vs. immersion technique 10
Conventional IOL power calculation formulae 89
Conventional keratometers 86, 129
   measure 27
Conventional keratometry
   devices 19
   techniques 47
Conventional simulated keratometry 19
Conventional ultrasonic methods 42
Conversion factors 136
Convexo-concave 138
Cornea-based refractive surgical procedures 85
Corneal ablative procedures 85
Corneal apex, decentered 126*f*
Corneal astigmatism undergo 134
Corneal bypass method 88
Corneal cross-linking 124
Corneal curvature 39, 134
   and power 26*fc*
   increase 135
   measurement of 19, 101
Corneal diameter 36, 39, 41
Corneal ectasia 29, 30, 121
Corneal ectatic disorders 121
Corneal indentation 12
Corneal pathology 121
Corneal plane
   myopic correction in 90
   refractive correction at 98
Corneal power 19, 20, 22
   and curvature 47
   effective 93, 95
   estimation, Scheimpflug tomography for 95
   measurement 20*t*, 29, 30*t*, 102
      technique for 30
   methods to calculate 19
   postoperative 90, 93
Corneal radius 98
   corrected 98
Corneal scars 29, 30, 43, 129
Corneal surface
   anterior 23
   posterior 23
Corneal thickness 124
Corneal tomography 28
   devices 19, 41
Corneal topographers measure 86
Corneal topography, placido disk-based 27
Corneal WF analysis 34, 37
Corrected refractive index, postoperative 90
Counseling 123
Cryotherapy 135
Crystalline lens power 112
Curvature, postoperative radius of 90

D

Dense cataract 15
Descemet membrane endothelial keratoplasty 30
Descemet stripping
   automated endothelial keratoplasty 127
   endothelial keratoplasty 30
Diameter hexagonal pattern 39
Document stability 123
Domain optical coherence tomography 33
Donzis-Kastle-Gordon formula 57
Double-K
   method 89
   modified methods 89
   no-history method 94

E

Early theoretical formulas 3
Ectasia 123
Effective lens position, estimation of 6
Emmetropia verifying optical 62
Encircling band 134
Endothelial keratoplasty 29, 30, 128
Epiretinal membrane 16, 134
Equivalent keratometry reading 20, 22, 29, 30, 93, 96, 125*f*
Extensive segmental buckling 135
Extreme gradient boosting 75
Eye 141*fc*, 148
   acquiring scans in 44
   rubbing, chronic 121
   undergoing simultaneous penetrating
      keratoplasty 120

F

Feiz-Mannis IOL power adjustment method 88
Fellow eye axial length 137
Final adjusted anterior central corneal power 90

Five-variable vergence formulae 64
Formula error 86, 102
Fourier domain interferometry 35
Fourteen methods 97

G

Galilei dual Scheimpflug analyzer 25
Galilei G6 42, 96
Gas tamponade, fffect of 139
Gaussian optics 19, 61
   thick-lens formula 21, 22
   thin-lens formulae 68, 69*t*
Gills' nomogram 160*t*
Good quality A-scan 12*f*
   characteristics of 11

H

Haigis and Super Ladas formula 63
Haigis formula 64
   utilizes 64
Haigis-L formula 94
Haptic-to-haptic diameter 156
Hill refractive vergence formula 159
Hill-radial basis function 3.0 76
Hill-RBF 3.0 76
Hoffer Q formula 63, 149
   incorporates 63
Hoffer Q/Savini/Taroni 79
Holladay 1 formula 63
Holladay 2 formula 65, 103
Holladay R formula 159
Human eye, normal development of 112
Hyperopia, residual 160
Hyperopic prediction error 140
Hyperopic predictive errors, prevent 151

I

Immersion A-scan 10*f*
Immersion technique 10, 11
Implantable collamer lens 104
Individual refractive index 41
Instrument 49
   error 86, 102, 122
   to assess corneal curvature 23*t*
   to measure corneal power 22
Integrated biometers 36
Interferogram 37
Interpreting A-scan 11
Intraocular lens 3, 6, 13, 25, 49, 50, 62, 69, 88, 90, 122, 124, 156, 157, 159-161
   aspheric 71
   choice of 104, 127, 128, 138
   constant 62
      optimization of 65, 140

cylinder power, effective 50
design 139
   related factors 150
diameter 157
first 3, 61
formula 98
high powered 148
implantation 115*t*
   secondary piggyback 159
multifocal 127
optical methods for 68
premium 52*f*
related factors 149
scleral-fixated 158, 161
secondary 156
specific 93
sulcus-fixated 160
toric 71
type of 139
Intraocular lens power 98, 112, 138, 142, 143, 156, 160
   adjustment 89, 158, 161, 161*t*
      sliding scale for 161*t*
   calculation 5, 47, 52*f*, 65, 66, 75, 76*t*, 83, 85, 101, 103, 112, 116, 121, 122*t*, 123, 124*fc*, 125, 127, 129, 134, 135, 138, 140, 148, 150, 159
      challenges in 138, 140
   error in 85, 102
   evolution of 1, 3
   method 86, 87*f*, 88*t*, 90*t*, 91, 92*t*, 99, 99*t*, 100-102
   numerical ray-tracing software for 70
   planning 150*fc*, 152*fc*
   prerequisites before 123
   calculation formula 38*f*, 39-41, 55, 57, 62, 76, 77*t*, 122
      evolution of 3, 4*f*
      new-generation 80
      ray-tracing based 70*t*
   formula 6, 66, 103, 113
      calculates 4
      generations of 6*t*
   ranging, reduction in 160
   residual 159
   undercorrection 115
Intraoperative aberrometry 71, 72, 100, 103
   measurements 72
IOLMaster 700 16*f*, 40
Iris-claw
   intraocular lens 157
   lenses 157*t*
      retropupillary implantation of 157
Iris-fixated intraocular lens 157
Irregular corneas, power calculation in 121
Irregular tear film 122

J

Javal and Schiotz keratometer 26

K

Kane formula 77, 78
Keratoconus 122*t*, 124*fc*, 126*f*
Keratometer 22, 26
Keratometric index error 85, 102
Keratometry 19, 20, 30, 37, 62, 70, 88, 90, 93, 98, 100, 122, 124, 161
   adjusted 89
   estimation 128
   measurement 5, 6, 39
   methods using 91, 95
   minimal effect of 151
   mode of 23-25
   postoperative 88-90, 98
   preoperative 49*t*, 88, 90
   readings 19
      centered 126*f*
   values 22-25
Keratopathy 43
Keratoplasty 127

L

Ladas super formula 2.0 64, 77, 78
Lamellar keratoplasty 128
   anterior 128
Laser
   interference biometry 66
   interferometry based optical biometers 14
   vision correction 70
Laser-assisted in situ keratomileusis 52, 85, 100
Lens
   position, effective 3, 5, 6, 30, 68, 69, 75, 86, 90, 122, 148
   thickness 6, 36, 37, 62, 69, 70, 76, 130, 136
Lenstar LS 900 23, 27, 33, 39, 69
Light-emitting diode 49
Long eyes 150
   appropriate formula in 151, 149
   error in 150
Lower refractive index 138

M

Macular edema 16, 134
Maloney method 91
   modified 91
Manifest refraction, change in 90
Manual keratometers 26*t*, 124
Manual keratometry 49
Masket formula 100
Masket method, modified 100
Mean pupil power 21, 93
Michelson interferometer 37
Modern-day refractive surgery, armamentarium of 85
Modern-day vergence formulae 61, 62
Moiré pattern 72
Multimode laser diode infrared radiation 37
Myopia, residual 160
Myopic laser-assisted in situ keratomileusis 98*t*
Myopic prediction error 140
Myopic shift 139, 141

O

OA 2000 41
Ocular biometric data 160
Oil-filled eyes 136, 136*t*, 138
Olsen formula 68-70
Optical biometers 14, 23, 27, 33, 37, 38, 40, 42, 113, 138
   different 43
   incorporated 41
   over ultrasonic
      biometry, disadvantages of 43
      methods, advantages of 42
   types of 33, 34*t*
Optical biometry 13, 14, 33, 103, 141
   methods 9
   preoperative user adjusted 142
   technology in 44
Optical coherence tomography 13, 15, 20, 25, 40, 47, 49, 100, 124, 139
   based device 25
   based methods 95
Optical length 37
Optical low coherence
   interferometry 34, 36, 40
   reflectometry 13, 33, 34, 36
      based optical biometers 39
Optima 157

P

Pars plana vitrectomy 138
Partial coherence interferometry 13, 33, 34, 36
   optical biometer 96
Pediatric cataract
   management of 112
   surgery 114
Pediatric piggyback intraocular lens calculator 116, 159
Pentacam (Oculus Optikgeräte) 24, 29
Pentacam AXL (oculus) 42
Peripheral corneal relaxing incision 50
Phakic intraocular lens 103
   implantation 85
Photorefractive keratectomy 52, 85, 98*t*, 100
Piggyback intraocular lens 156, 159
   implantation, refractive outcomes of 160, 161
   power calculation 160*t*
Placido disk topography 37
   applications of 28
Polymethyl methacrylate 138

Polypseudophakia
    primary 159
        residual power in 159*t*
    temporary 116
Poor visual acuity 134
Post-corneal refractive surgery 87*fc*
Post-endothelial keratoplasty 30
Posterior chamber phakic intraocular lens 103
Posterior corneal
    apex 70
    steepening 128
    surface 23
Posterior corneal astigmatism 47, 47*t*, 48, 52*f*
    estimation of 50
Posterior corneal curvature 22, 37, 47-49, 125*f*
    assessment of 48*fc*
    measurement of 20, 48, 49, 95
Post-hyperopic corneal ablative procedures 86
Post-laser
    refractive surgery patients 99*t*
    vision correction 71
Post-myopic corneal laser ablative surgery 30
Post-radial keratotomy 30, 102
Post-refractive surgery 31, 38
    intraocular lens power calculation 85
Post-smile patients 101
Post-vitrectomized eyes 142
Potvin-Shammas-Hill formula 96
Prager shell 10*f*
Pre-cataract surgery parameters 104, 107, 143
Pre-pupillary fixation 157*t*
Prerefractive surgery spherical equivalent 90
Previtrectomy axial length 138
Probe gently touching cornea 10*f*
Probe tip fixation light 10*f*
Progressive vision loss 121
Pseudophakic patients 160, 161
Pseudophakic pediatric eyes, refractive growth in 112
Pupil diameter 37
Pupillary diameter 36, 41

R

Radial basis function 49, 77
Radial keratotomy 52, 102
Radius
    correcting factor 93
    error 86, 102
    of curvature, preoperative 90
    posterior 70
Ray tracing 97
    formula 4, 68, 69, 69*t*, 71
        estimate 71
        principle of 68
    method 21, 68, 71, 97, 128
    software 100
Refracting surface 68

Refraction
    based methods 91
    error, index of 122
    index of 70
    residual 5
Refractive change, surgically induced 88-90, 100
Refractive correction, magnitude of 89, 90
Refractive error 88
    and biometry 161
    calculation, target 89
    postoperative 114, 115*t*
Refractive goal, postoperative 114
Refractive growth 112
Refractive index 20, 61
    methods, adjusted 89
    theoretical variable 93
Refractive outcomes, methods to improve 140, 141
Refractive power, effective 90, 98
Refractive prediction error 117
Refractive status 134
Refractive vergence formula 160
Regression analysis 57
Regression formulae 4, 57, 59
    limitations of 59
    relevance of 59
Retina 148
Retinal detachment 15, 141
    phacovitrectomy for 140
Retinal pathologies 139
Retinal pigment epithelium 37, 141
Retinal visualization, enhanced 41
Retropupillary fixation 157, 157*t*
Retropupillary implantation 157
Retropupillary space 157
Retrosilicone space 136
Rhegmatogenous retinal detachment 134, 141*fc*
Right eye 104
    cataract surgery 106

S

Sanders-Retzlaff-Kraff formula 57, 58
    modifications of 58
Sanders-Retzlaff-Kraff theoretic 77
Savini method 91
Scheimpflug imaging 48
    based devices 24
Scheimpflug topography (pentacam) 125*f*
Scheimpflug-based devices 44, 128
Scleral buckle 134, 134*t*, 135
    presence of 134
Seitz method 88
Seven-variable vergence formula 65
Shammas-PL formula 94
Short eyes 148
    error in 148
Signal to noise ratio 141

Silicone oil 134
   filled eyes 15, 16, 135
   removal 135, 138
Simulated keratometry 20, 25, 30
   postoperative 90, 93
   preoperative 90
   values 91
      modifications of 91
Simultaneous cataract surgery 135
   refractive outcomes of 136
Sirius anterior segment evaluation system combines 96
Sirius topographer 24
Slight hyperopic target refraction 140
Small incision lenticule extraction 85
Snell's law 21, 68
Speicher method 88
Spherical aberration 70
Spherical equivalent 93
   postoperative 160
   refractive error 93
SRK-T formula 63
Standard error 137
Staphyloma, posterior 15, 16
Sulcus intraocular lens
   implantation during cataract surgery 161t
   power adjustment for 159, 161
Super Ladas formula 64
Super luminescent diode 37
Surgical techniques 140
Swept source optical coherence tomography optical biometer 16f

T

Talbot-Moiré interferometry 72
Thick-lens model considers 62
Thijssen's formula 3
Thin-lens
   model, paraxial formulae based on 69
   paraxial formula 19
   principles of 19
Third-generation formulae 86
Three-variable vergence formulae 63
Tomographic methods 103
Total corneal
   power 20, 21, 93, 96, 98
   refractive power 20, 21, 24, 29, 30, 36, 93, 96
Total keratometry 22, 95, 100
   prediction formulae for 50

Total laser
   correction, spherical equivalent of 90
   treatment 89
True net power 20, 21, 36, 93, 96, 98, 125
True refractive vitreal index 140
Two-variable vergence formulae 62

U

Ultrasonic biometry, techniques of 11t
Ultrasonic methods 136
Ultrasound beam, misalignment of 12
Ultrasound biometry
   error in 12
   measurements using 9
   techniques of 9

V

Van der Heijde's formula 3
Vergence formula 4, 61, 62, 62t
   drawbacks of 66
   principle of 61
Verisyse intraocular lens 157
Vernal keratoconjunctivitis 121
Vertex distance 5
Vertex-centered measurements 126f
Vision loss, cause of 123
Visual acuity, uncorrected 161
Visual axis opacities 43
Vitreomacular traction 16
Vitreoretinal interface abnormalities 15, 16
Vitreous
   cavity 136
   hemorrhage 43
   with aqueous, replacement of 139

W

Wang Koch Maloney method 91, 94
Wang method 91
Wang-Koch
   adjustment 65
   modification 64
White-to-white corneal diameter 157t

Z

ZEISS artificial intelligence intraocular lens calculator 78
Ziemer ophthalmic systems 42, 95

EU GSPR Authorised Reprsentative
Logos Europe, 9 rue Nicolas Poussin
1700, La Rochelle, France
Phone: +33 (0) 6 67 93 73 78
E-mail: contact@logoseurope.eu

www.ingramcontent.com/pod-product-compliance
Ingram Content Group UK Ltd.
Pitfield, Milton Keynes, MK11 3LW, UK
UKHW050135060725
460398UK00019B/20